# HAND CLINICS

## Pediatric Fractures, Dislocations, and Sequelae

GUEST EDITOR
Scott H. Kozin, MD

February 2006 • Volume 22 • Number 1

**SAUNDERS**

An Imprint of Elsevier, Inc.
PHILADELPHIA   LONDON   TORONTO   MONTREAL   SYDNEY   TOKYO

**W.B. SAUNDERS COMPANY**
*A Division of Elsevier Inc.*

1600 John F. Kennedy Blvd. • Suite 1800 • Philadelphia, Pennsylvania 19103

http://www.theclinics.com

**HAND CLINICS**
**February 2006**
Editor: Debora Dellapena

Volume 22, Number 1
ISSN 0749-0712
ISBN 1-4160-3506-0

The ideas and opinions expressed in *Hand Clinics* do not necessarily reflect those of the Publisher. The Publisher does not assume any responsibility for any injury and/or damage to persons or property arising out of or related to any use of the material contained in this periodical. The reader is advised to check the appropriate medical literature and the product information provided by the manufacturer of each drug to be administered to verify the dosage, the method and duration of administration, or contraindications. It is the responsibility of the treating physician or other health care professional, relying on independent experience and knowledge of the patient, to determine drug dosages and the best treatment for the patient. Mention of any product in this issue should not be construed as endorsement by the contributors, editors, or the Publisher of the product or manufacturers' claims.

*Hand Clinics* (ISSN 0749-0712) is published quarterly by W.B. Saunders, 360 Park Avenue South, New York, NY 10010-1710. Months of publication are February, May, August, and November. Business and Editorial Offices: 1600 John F. Kennedy Blvd., Suite 1800, Philadelphia, PA 19103-2899. Accounting and Circulation Offices: 6277 Sea Harbor Drive, Orlando, FL 32887-4800. Periodicals postage paid at New York, NY, and additional mailing offices. Subscription price is $215.00 per year (U.S. individuals), $335.00 per year (U.S. institutions), $110.00 per year (US students), $245.00 per year (Canadian individuals), $375.00 per year (Canadian institutions), $135.00 (Canadian students), $275.00 per year (international individuals), $375.00 per year (international institutions), and $135.00 per year (international students). Foreign air speed delivery is included in all *Clinics* subscription prices. All prices are subject to change without notice. POSTMASTER: Send address changes to *Hand Clinics*, Elsevier Periodicals Customer Service, 6277 Sea Harbor Drive, Orlando, FL 32887-4800. **Customer Service: 1-800-654-2452 (US). From outside the US, call 1-407-345-4000. E-mail: hhspcs@harcourt.com.**

Reprints. For copies of 100 or more, of articles in this publication, please contact the Commercial Rights Department, Elsevier Inc., 360 Park Avenue South, New York, NY 10010-1710. Tel: (212) 633-3813, Fax: (212) 462-1935, e-mail: reprints@elsevier.com

*Hand Clinics* is covered in *Index Medicus, Current Contents/Clinical Medicine, EMBASE/Excerpta Medica,* and *ISI/BIOMED.*

Printed in the United States of America.

# GUEST EDITOR

**SCOTT H. KOZIN, MD,** Associate Professor of Orthopaedic Surgery, Temple University; Hand Surgeon, Shriners Hospitals for Children, Philadelphia, Pennsylvania

# CONTRIBUTORS

**DONALD S. BAE, MD,** Instructor in Orthopaedic Surgery, Harvard Medical School; Associate in Orthopaedic Surgery, Children's Hospital, Boston, Massachusetts

**MARK BARATZ, MD,** Director, Division of Hand and Upper Extremity Surgeries, Allegheny Orthopedic Associates, Allegheny General Hospital, Pittsburgh, Pennsylvania

**BENJAMIN CHANG, MD, FACS,** Division of Plastic Surgery, The Children's Hospital of Philadelphia; Associate Professor of Clinical Surgery, University of Pennsylvania, Philadelphia, Pennsylvania

**ROGER CORNWALL, MD,** Pediatric Hand and Upper Extremity Surgeon, The Children's Hospital of Philadelphia; Assistant Professor of Orthopaedic Surgery, University of Pennsylvania School of Medicine, Philadelphia, Pennsylvania

**BASSEM T. ELHASSAN, MD,** Hand Fellow, Department of Orthopedic Surgery, Division of Hand Surgery, Mayo Medical College, Rochester, Minnesota

**GLORIA R. GOGOLA, MD,** Assistant Professor, Department of Orthopaedics, University of Texas Health Science Center, Houston, Texas

**MARTIN J. HERMAN, MD,** Associate Professor of Orthopedic Surgery, Division of Orthopedic Surgery, Drexel University College of Medicine, St. Christopher's Hospital for Children, Philadelphia, Pennsylvania

**HARISH S. HOSALKAR, MD, MBMS (Orth),** Division of Orthopedic Surgery, The Children's Hospital of Philadelphia, Philadelphia, Pennsylvania

**JOSEPH KHOURY, MD,** Shriners Hospitals for Children, Erie, Pennsylvania

**L. ANDREW KOMAN, MD,** Professor and Vice Chair, Director of Hand Surgery Fellowship, Department of Orthopaedic Surgery, Wake Forest University, School of Medicine, Winston-Salem, North Carolina

**SCOTT H. KOZIN, MD,** Associate Professor of Orthopaedic Surgery, Temple University; Hand Surgeon, Shriners Hospitals for Children, Philadelphia, Pennsylvania

**ZHONGYU LI, MD, PhD,** Assistant Professor, Department of Orthopaedic Surgery, Wake Forest University, School of Medicine, Winston-Salem, North Carolina

**JOHN D. LUBAHN, MD,** Hamot Medical Center, Erie, Pennsylvania

**SILAS T. MARSHALL, BA,** Student of Medicine, Drexel University College of Medicine, Philadelphia, Pennsylvania

**JONAS L. MATZON, MD,** Division of Orthopedic Surgery, The Children's Hospital of Philadelphia, Philadelphia, Pennsylvania

**CHAD MICUCCI, MD,** Allegheny Orthopedic Associates, Allegheny General Hospital, Pittsburgh, Pennsylvania

**ANASTASIOS PAPADONIKOLAKIS, MD,** Resident, Department of Orthopaedic Surgery, Wake Forest University, School of Medicine, Winston-Salem, North Carolina

**MARK SANGIMINO, MD,** Allegheny Orthopedic Associates, Allegheny General Hospital, Pittsburgh, Pennsylvania

**FRANCES SHARPE, MD,** Orthopedic Surgeon, Southern California Permanente Medical Group, Fontana, California

**ALEXANDER Y. SHIN, MD,** Consultant and Associate Professor, Department of Orthopedic Surgery, Division of Hand Surgery, Mayo Medical College, Rochester, Minnesota

**BETH P. SMITH, PhD,** Associate Professor, Department of Orthopaedic Surgery, Wake Forest University, School of Medicine, Winston-Salem, North Carolina

**MILAN STEVANOVIC, MD,** Professor of Orthopedics and Surgery, University of Southern California Keck School of Medicine, Los Angeles, California

**SHAWN W. STORM, DO,** Hamot Medical Center, Erie, Pennsylvania

**ANN VANHEEST, MD,** Associate Professor, Department of Orthopaedic Surgery, University of Minnesota, Minneapolis; Gillette Children's Specialtycare Hospital, St. Paul; Shriner's Hospital for Children-Twin Cities Unit, Minneapolis, Minnesota

**PETER M. WATERS, MD,** Professor in Orthopaedic Surgery, Harvard Medical School; Director, Hand and Upper Extremity Program, Children's Hospital, Boston, Massachusetts

**D. PATRICK WILLIAMS, DO,** Hamot Medical Center, Erie, Pennsylvania

# CONTENTS

> Metacarpal fractures in the finger rays are common injuries in children's hands. Fractures of the finger metacarpals account for 10% to 39% of all hand fractures in children, especially in the 13- to 16-year age group. Most of these fractures can be treated successfully nonoperatively, although a subset requires more aggressive treatment. Results following appropriate care of these fractures are generally good, although complications can occur. This article reviews fractures and dislocations involving the finger metacarpals in children, provides standard treatment algorithms, and highlights potential pitfalls in their management.

> Phalangeal fractures in children are common, and conservative treatment leads frequently to a good functional outcome. Articular or displaced fractures require early recognition and special attention, including surgery. In children, remodeling occurs primarily in the sagittal plane, and rotational deformities are often unacceptable.

> The pediatric hand thumb is vulnerable to injury for several reasons. Young children inadvertently place their thumbs in vulnerable positions, such as doors and drawers. Adolescents participate in sporting recreational events, such as skiing, bike riding, or motorcycle riding, that require the thumb to participate in firm grasp. Skiing or biking mishaps frequently result in injury to the thumb. In children, fractures and fracture-dislocations are more common than true dislocations, because the bone is more fragile than the ligaments.

> Scaphoid fractures are uncommon in the pediatric age group and misdiagnosis is common secondary to the rarity of this injury. Overall scaphoid fractures in children

have a better prognosis when compared with adult scaphoid fractures. Most pediatric scaphoid fractures can be treated with cast immobilization, which results in union and a return to normal activities. Nonunion is uncommon and treatment options include further immobilization, percutaneous bone grafting, or open reduction and internal fixation with or without bone grafting. These treatments uniformly result in scaphoid union in the vast majority of cases.

reduction, and palsies that develop after fracture reduction. For closed fractures associated with nerve palsy at the time of initial injury, observation and serial examination after reduction is recommended. If there is no return of nerve function on examination or electrodiagnostic testing by 4 months, operative exploration is indicated.

# FORTHCOMING ISSUES

# RECENT ISSUES

ELSEVIER
SAUNDERS

Hand Clin 22 (2006) ix–x

Preface

# Pediatric Fractures, Dislocations, and Sequelae

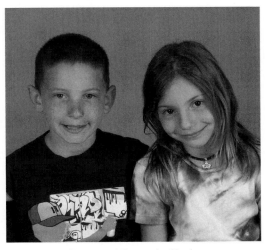

Bryan and Samantha Kozin

Children (like our kids pictured above) have particular characteristics that make them special. Kids are not small adults, and pediatric fractures are different than adult fractures. Children have a propensity to injury their upper extremities. Young children inadvertently place their limbs in untoward positions, such as doors and drawers. Adolescents participate in sporting recreational events, such as skiing, bike riding, or gymnastics that frequently result in injury. Fractures can occur about the hand, wrist, forearm, and elbow. Diagnosis is complicated by the lack of ossification and the difficulties of examining a child. This issue of the *Hand Clinics* is devoted to pediatric fractures, dislocations, and their complications—an arduous task.

In attempt to accomplish this enterprise, an outstanding array of experts in pediatric upper extremity was assembled. The authors possess extensive knowledge in their particular assignment. The goal was to cover fractures from the fingertips to the elbow with a focus on treatments and complications. The hand is covered by a series of articles that deals with fractures and

dislocations about the phalanges, interphalangeal joints, metacarpophalangeal joints, and metacarpals. The carpus and wrist articles focuses on the scaphoid with its increasing prevalence and advancing treatment algorithms. In addition, distal radius fractures and triangular fibrocartilage tears are discussed in a separate article devoted solely to this topic.

Moving up the forearm and elbow, the treatment of the pediatric forearm fracture is controversial and the management is evolving over time. Therefore, an article was included devoted to the indications and technique of intramedullary nailing. Moving upward to the elbow, pediatric elbow fractures remain a vexing problem for physicians. Consequently, a sequence of articles was incorporated that discuss medial condylar, lateral condylar, and supracondylar fractures.

Despite our best efforts, complications occur after pediatric upper extremity fractures. As a result, an entire section was devoted to the recognition and management of these problems. Acute neurovascular problems are covered in articles on nerve palsies and Volkman's ischemic contracture.

Chronic problems are discussed in articles that discuss with wrist and elbow deformities after fracture.

I would like to thank all the contributors for their timely submission of superb manuscripts. In addition, this issue of the *Hand Clinics* required the diligent effort of Deb Dellapena at Elsevier. Lastly, I would like to thank kids for being kids; they make my job more wonderful and our adult life more pleasurable.

Scott H. Kozin, MD
*Shriners Hospitals for Children*
*3551 North Broad Street*
*Philadelphia, PA 19140, USA*

*E-mail address:* skozin@shrinenet.org

# Finger Metacarpal Fractures and Dislocations in Children

### Roger Cornwall, MD[a,b,*]

[a]*The Children's Hospital of Philadelphia, Division of Orthopaedics, Wood Center, 2nd Floor,
34th Street and Civic Center Boulevard, Philadelphia, PA 19104, USA*
[b]*Orthopaedic Surgery, University of Pennsylvania School of Medicine, Philadelphia, PA 19104, USA*

Metacarpal fractures in the finger rays are common injuries in children's hands. Fractures of the finger metacarpals account for 10% to 39% of all hand fractures in children [1–4], especially in the 13- to 16-year age group [3]. Most of these fractures can be treated successfully nonoperatively, although a subset requires more aggressive treatment. Results following appropriate care of these fractures are generally good, although complications can occur. This article reviews fractures and dislocations involving the finger metacarpals in children, provides standard treatment algorithms, and highlights potential pitfalls in their management.

## Metacarpal base fractures and carpometacarpal dislocations

Fractures at the bases of the finger metacarpal fractures account for 13% to 20% of finger metacarpal fractures in children, with one half to two thirds occurring in the small finger ray [2,3]. Dislocations of the finger carpometacarpal (CMC) joints are rare in children, and the literature on this topic is limited mostly to case reports [5–7]. Nonetheless, the two injuries can coexist, especially in the small finger ray, where an intra-articular metacarpal base fracture can allow subluxation or dislocation of the CMC joint analogous to a Bennett fracture in the thumb [6]. Most metacarpal base fractures are transverse in fracture pattern

and likely result from axial loading of a flexed metacarpal. This theory may explain the higher incidence of metacarpal base fractures in the small finger ray, which has the most mobile CMC joint. Crush injuries can cause metacarpal base fractures also, and it is wise to suspect a high-energy mechanism of injury in these fractures (Fig. 1).

Evaluation of patients who have fractures of the metacarpal bases should include a careful assessment of swelling and neurovascular status, because compartment syndrome of the hand can accompany these injuries, especially if multiple rays are injured or if the mechanism of injury was a crush (Fig. 2). Examination may not reveal a visible or palpable deformity even in displaced fractures or CMC dislocations because of the abundant swelling dorsally. Examination for rotational malalignment is important, although the flexion of the fingers necessary for determining rotational alignment may be difficult because of severe swelling.

Radiographic evaluation of metacarpal base and CMC injuries may be challenging. An adequate lateral view of each ray is required, and because of the transverse arch of the metacarpals, multiple oblique views may be required. Computed tomography may be helpful in some cases, such as in assessing intra-articular metacarpal base fractures or suspected adjacent carpal fractures.

Nondisplaced or minimally displaced extra-articular fractures of the metacarpal bases generally can be treated conservatively with closed immobilization. If considerable swelling exists, splints should be used initially rather than casts, and the child should be monitored closely for signs of impending compartment syndrome. As

* The Children's Hospital of Philadelphia, Division of Orthopaedics, Wood Center, 2nd Floor, 34th Street and Civic Center Boulevard, Philadelphia, PA 19104.
*E-mail address:* cornwall@email.chop.edu

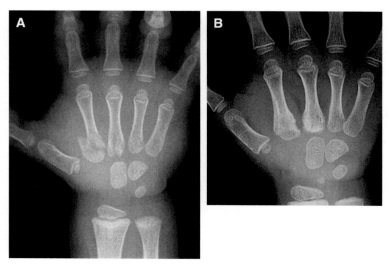

Fig. 1. (*A*) Anteroposterior radiograph of a 3-year-old child whose hand was crushed by a fence gate, producing fractures of the index and middle finger metacarpal bases. (*B*) Remodeling was complete at 5 months following nonoperative fracture treatment.

swelling abates, splints or casts should be adjusted. Metacarpal base fractures heal reliably, and typically require only 3 to 4 weeks of immobilization followed by active range of motion exercises with activity restriction for an additional 2 weeks.

Displaced metacarpal base fractures and dislocations of the CMC joints generally can be reduced by closed means. Although regional anesthesia in the form of a wrist block can provide adequate analgesia, young children often require conscious sedation or general anesthesia because of anxiety. Reduction is accomplished using longitudinal traction on the involved rays coupled with a volarly directed pressure on the displaced metacarpal base (in a dorsal CMC dislocation) or metacarpal shaft (in a dorsally displaced metacarpal base fracture). Rotational malalignment should be corrected by flexing the metacarpophalangeal (MCP) joint 90° to tighten the MCP collateral ligaments and then using the proximal phalanx segment as a rotational lever arm. In

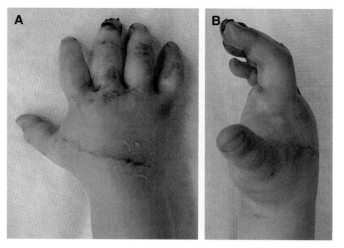

Fig. 2. (*A*) Frontal and (*B*) lateral clinical photographs of the child pictured in Fig. 1. Note severe swelling, including convexity of the palm. Compartment pressures were found to be elevated and emergent fasciotomies were performed.

some instances reduction of a CMC dislocation cannot be achieved by closed means, and open reduction is required [7]. A longitudinal dorsal incision over the involved joint or over the interspace between two adjacent involved joints provides good exposure to the dislocated joint and involved articular surfaces. Longitudinal incisions can be continued distally for interosseus fasciotomies if necessary.

Once a displaced, extra-articular metacarpal base fracture has been reduced by closed or open means, stability should be assessed. Fluoroscopy is particularly helpful in determining success and stability of reduction. Transverse metacarpal base fractures are typically stable following closed reduction and can be immobilized in a splint or cast (if swelling allows) for 3 to 4 weeks.

Conversely, CMC dislocations and fracture-dislocations are typically unstable, and casts are usually insufficient for maintaining an anatomic joint reduction owing to the abundant dorsal swelling that prohibits adequate molding of the cast. Percutaneous pinning therefore is advocated for CMC dislocations [8,9]. In an isolated small finger CMC dislocation, transverse pins through the metacarpal base into the adjacent metacarpal bases may be adequate, although oblique pins placed through the metacarpal base and across the CMC joint are also useful. In dislocations of multiple rays, transverse pins are not sufficient and oblique pins are difficult to introduce, especially in the central rays. In these cases, pins can be introduced distally at the collateral recesses and driven proximally through the intramedullary canal and across the reduced CMC joint [5,9]. This technique is technically challenging, and care must be taken to avoid injury to the metacarpal physes during pin introduction. The pins are left out of the skin but are protected under a well-padded splint or cast. The pins are pulled in the office or clinic after 5 to 6 weeks in the case of a dislocation or 4 weeks in the case of an unstable fracture, provided adequate bony union is evident radiographically. Active and passive range of motion exercises are begun with activity limitation until full range of motion has been achieved. Associated soft tissue injury or compartment syndrome may slow rehabilitation, and formal hand therapy may be required.

## Metacarpal shaft fractures

Fractures of the finger metacarpal shafts are not common in children. In two series, [2,3], metacarpal shaft fractures accounted for 10% to 14% of finger metacarpal fractures and 3% to 5% of hand fractures overall. These fractures were nearly evenly distributed among the middle, ring, and small rays, with no index metacarpal shaft fractures reported in either series. Most metacarpal shaft fractures are spiral in pattern [3], indicating a torsional mechanism of injury. Transverse fractures occur less frequently and represent bending forces, such as may occur when a hand is stepped on in a football pile-up [9].

Clinical examination of a child's hand with a metacarpal shaft fracture may reveal considerable swelling dorsally that obscures sagittal plane deformities. Rotational deformities are common, especially in spiral fractures, so clinical examination must include a careful evaluation of rotation. As with metacarpal base fractures, high-energy injuries causing multiple fractures may be associated with compartment syndrome, so a careful clinical examination is important.

Nondisplaced metacarpal shaft fractures can be treated by closed immobilization. Casts are preferred over splints, if swelling allows, because splints are removed easily by children and adolescents. Metacarpal shaft fractures can be slower to heal than those at the base or neck of the metacarpal, and immobilization should be continued for 4 to 6 weeks or until radiographs demonstrate sufficient healing. Stiffness is not typically a problem in children and adolescents who have metacarpal shaft fractures treated nonoperatively.

Most displaced metacarpal shaft fractures in children and adolescents are amenable to closed reduction and most are stable enough to allow cast immobilization after reduction [9]. Rotational control can be ensured by flexing the MCP joints and buddy-taping adjacent fingers inside the cast. Flexion deformity can be controlled with a well-molded cast or splint. Radiographs should be obtained after cast placement to ensure adequate reduction and well-located molding. The fracture may displace within the cast, especially as swelling subsides, so follow-up radiographs should be obtained at 1 and 2 weeks to ensure maintenance of reduction. Immobilization should be continued for 4 to 6 weeks or until radiographs demonstrate adequate healing.

Some metacarpal shaft fractures are not amenable to cast immobilization. Long oblique or spiral fractures have a tendency to shorten, and this displacement cannot be controlled adequately with a cast or splint. Also, multiple metacarpal shaft fractures can be unstable and require more aggressive treatment. For single unstable meta-carpal shaft fractures, percutaneous pinning works well. Transverse fractures can be controlled with transverse pins securing the proximal and distal fragments to adjacent stable metacarpals (Fig. 3). Two pins in the distal fragment and one pin in the proximal fragment suffice. Alternatively, intramedullary fixation can be used with Kirschner wires inserted through the collateral recesses. Care must be taken to avoid injury to the physes through such an approach. Long oblique or spiral fractures that are unstable can be controlled with interfragmentary pins or screws, although the latter requires open reduction with its attendant risks. Plate fixation is not needed often but may be used for multiple adjacent transverse fractures. If internal fixation with screws or plates is used, stiffness may develop from tendon adhesions, and motion should be started as soon as allowed by the stability of the fixation and the healing of the fracture. If percutaneous pins are used, they are left in place for 5 to 6 weeks, given the slower healing of the metacarpal shafts. If internal fixation is used, the plates/screws may need to be removed for tendon irritation.

## Metacarpal neck fractures

Fractures of the metacarpal neck account for 56% to 70% of all finger metacarpal fractures in children [2,3]. Small finger metacarpal neck fractures are the most common and account for 41% to 80% of all metacarpal fractures [2–4]. Similarly, small finger metacarpal neck fractures are the second most common hand fracture in children overall [2,3] and the most common hand fracture in the 13- to 16-year age group [3].

Most metacarpal neck fractures occur during conflict, especially in the adolescent age group. Falls and sporting injuries, however, can produce metacarpal neck fractures in younger children. Nonetheless, the mechanism of injury is typically axial loading and bending, producing transverse fractures with a typical apex–dorsal angulation. The fractures can involve the physis, but physeal fractures are discussed here separately.

Clinical evaluation of patients who have metacarpal neck fractures follows the principles of other metacarpal fractures. Rotation must be checked. Although swelling is generally prominent and may obscure flexion deformities, compartment syndrome is rare. Careful attention must be paid to overlying skin. Any break in the skin should raise suspicion for contamination of the fracture or MCP joint by a tooth. Competence of extensor tendons must be tested. Radiographic evaluation of metacarpal neck fractures is generally straightforward, although oblique views may be most helpful in determining displacement. One important note in determining displacement is noting the presence of pre-existing deformity from previous fracture. Combative adolescents may sustain several metacarpal neck fractures, and nondisplaced fractures can occur through previously malunited fractures (Fig. 4).

Metacarpal neck fractures can be nondisplaced, especially in younger children in whom the fracture pattern may be a simple buckle of the palmar cortex. Such fractures heal reliably in 3 to 4 weeks. Immobilization in a cast protects the tender fracture site from re-injury during healing and gives the parents peace of mind. Stiffness is

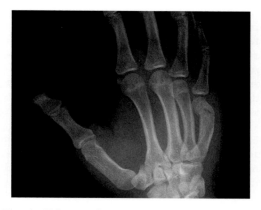

Fig. 4. Oblique radiograph demonstrating minimally displaced small finger metacarpal neck fracture through previously malunited and partially remodeled metacarpal neck fracture.

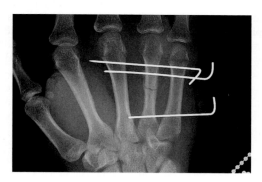

Fig. 3. Transverse percutaneous pinning construct for an unstable isolated metacarpal shaft fracture.

generally not a concern after cast immobilization in these young children.

Displaced metacarpal neck fractures usually are treated best with closed means. Debate exists regarding acceptable angulation of metacarpal neck fractures, although most agree that more angulation is acceptable in the small and ring finger rays than in the index and middle finger rays, and that younger patients who have remodeling potential can tolerate more angulation. Some investigators report remodeling of up to 70° of angulation [10], whereas others accept up to 30° to 35° of angulation in the ulnar two metacarpals and up to 10° to 20° in the index and middle rays [4,8]. The author generally agrees with the latter recommendation and accepts 10°, 20°, 30°, and 40° of angulation in the index through small finger metacarpals, respectively. These recommendations are for postreduction angulation. A small finger metacarpal neck fracture angulated 40° at presentation deserves an attempt at closed reduction. Rotational malalignment is not well tolerated and should be reduced.

Closed reduction of metacarpal neck fractures can be performed under wrist block or even hematoma block if the fracture occurred within 24 to 48 hours of presentation. Conscious sedation often is not needed for reduction, because children young enough to require sedation usually do not sustain widely displaced fractures. Reduction maneuvers are the same in children as in adults and include the Jahss maneuver [11] or simple three-point bending. Rotational alignment should be confirmed after reduction. Cast immobilization is preferred over splint treatment, if swelling allows, because splints generally are removed too easily by children and adolescents and often do not stay where they were placed even in compliant children (Fig. 5). Casts are left in place for 4 weeks or until clinical and radiographic union is achieved. Fractures requiring reduction are followed radiographically to ensure maintenance of reduction during healing, because fractures can redisplace as swelling subsides and the cast loosens.

An important consideration in cast treatment of reduced metacarpal neck fractures in children and adolescents is that the MCP joint can be immobilized safely at or near full extension. Such immobilization allows three-point molding at the fracture site, which is impossible when the MCP joint is flexed and the proximal phalanx obscures the palmar surface of the distal fragment. Stiffness is not a major concern in this patient population,

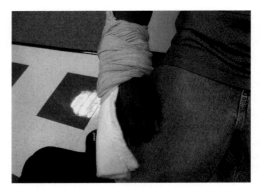

Fig. 5. Clinical photograph showing the typical fate of a splint applied following closed reduction of a metacarpal neck fracture in a child. The splint was removed by the patient immediately following reduction and then reapplied before presenting to the clinic for follow-up. Reduction had been lost. Casts are preferable to splints if swelling allows, given improved compliance.

and full range of motion generally is achieved within 1 to 2 weeks of cast removal without formal therapy.

Many patients who have substantially displaced metacarpal neck fractures present well after healing has begun. In such situations options include surgical reduction of the impending malunion or closed treatment and later osteotomy. The former is recommended for index and middle ray fractures in patients approaching skeletal maturity. The latter approach is acceptable in younger children, however, or those who have ring or small finger metacarpal neck fractures. Function in these patients ultimately may be good without the attendant risks of open reduction, and osteotomy may not be required.

Formal open reduction of metacarpal neck fractures rarely is needed, but fractures that are unstable after closed reduction, especially in the index and middle rays, may require percutaneous pin fixation. Pins can be inserted at the collateral recesses and crossed proximal to the fracture site. The MCP joint should be flexed during insertion to avoid tethering the collateral ligaments. After crossing the fracture site, the pins can be driven through the opposite cortex of the proximal fragment or driven down the medullary canal of the metacarpal. Either placement provides adequate resistance to flexion at the fracture site. Alternatively, pins can be placed transversely into the adjacent metacarpal neck or head. Such a technique avoids crossing the physis with pins and is helpful in fractures with inherent instability or comminution (Fig. 6). Pins are left out of the skin and are protected with a well-padded cast. Pins are pulled in the clinic at 4 weeks, after radiographs confirm adequate union.

Complications are uncommon following metacarpal neck fractures in children and adolescents. Stiffness is typically transient and formal therapy rarely is needed. Parents and patients should be made aware at the beginning of treatment of the cosmetic flattening of the knuckle that may be noticeable even in minimally angulated fractures. Refracture of the metacarpal neck may occur but likely is caused by persistent behavior patterns rather than osseus weakness.

## Metacarpal physeal and epiphyseal fractures

Fractures involving the finger metacarpal physes and epiphyses are uncommon. Mahabir and colleagues [2] found 13 finger metacarpal physeal fractures out of 72 finger metacarpal fractures (18%) and 185 hand fractures overall (7%). Although small finger metacarpal physeal fractures were the most common, extraphyseal metacarpal neck fractures outnumbered physeal fractures 3 to 1. Similarly in a series of 284 fractures of the finger metacarpals, Fischer and McElfresh [12] found 7% to involve the physis. Of these, 85% were Salter-Harris type II fractures analogous in mechanism of injury to metacarpal neck fractures. Hastings and Simmons found 20% of hand fractures to occur in metacarpals,

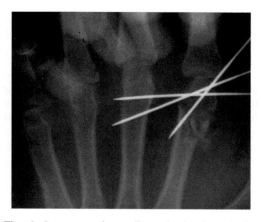

Fig. 6. Anteroposterior radiograph showing pinning technique for metacarpal neck fractures with considerable comminution, such as occurred in this adolescent victim of a gunshot wound. Pins can be placed across into adjacent metacarpals when insufficient bone exists at the metacarpal neck to provide stable pin fixation.

but only 8% of Salter-Harris type II fractures to occur in the metacarpals [1]. A possible explanation for the disproportionately low incidence of physeal fractures in the metacarpals compared with the phalanges is that the collateral ligaments at the finger MCP joints originate from the metacarpal epiphysis and metaphysis, stabilizing the physis [13].

Salter-Harris type II fractures of the finger metacarpals are treated in a manner analogous to extraphyseal metacarpal neck fractures. Late attempts at reduction should be avoided, however, to prevent additional injury to the growth plate. Although growth arrest is rare [14], displaced fractures should be followed radiographically until normal growth can be confirmed. Because most of such fractures occur in adolescents close to skeletal maturity, the potential for functional or cosmetic problems following growth arrest is low [12].

Epiphyseal fractures are rare in the skeletally immature finger metacarpal head. Fischer and McElfresh found two Salter-Harris type III fractures out of 284 finger metacarpal fractures [12]. Both were nondisplaced sagittal fractures and healed without complications. Prosser and Irvine [15] reported a nondisplaced transverse fracture of the metacarpal epiphysis, distal to the physes, that healed uneventfully. Others, however [8,16], have reported osteonecrosis of the metacarpal head following displaced epiphyseal fractures and postulated a causative effect of tamponade from an intra-articular effusion. Such a hypothesis has prompted some investigators to recommend considering aspiration of the MCP joint in the setting of an intra-articular fracture [8,9]. Nondisplaced fractures at the collateral ligament origin can be treated by closed means with casting until bony union or until asymptomatic, clinically stable fibrous union is achieved. Displaced epiphyseal fractures should be reduced, however, because articular congruity is important. Open reduction typically is required, and fixation can consist of smooth wires, screws, or sutures, depending on the size and location of the fragment (Fig. 7). In contrast to extra-articular metacarpal fractures, intra-articular fractures can cause persistent stiffness, pain, and dysfunction, even with optimal treatment.

## Metacarpophalangeal dislocations

The MCP joint is the most frequent site of dislocation in the child's hand [10,17,18]. Although most MCP dislocations occur in the

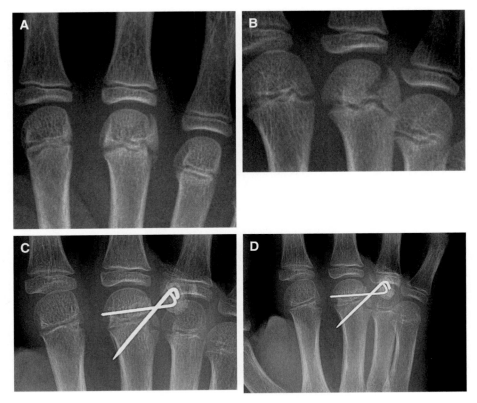

Fig. 7. (*A*) Anteroposterior and (*B*) oblique radiographs demonstrating a displaced metacarpal head fracture. (*C*) Anteroposterior and (*D*) oblique radiographs 4 weeks after open reduction and pin fixation.

thumb, dislocations in the index ray are the most often irreducible. The proximal phalanx typically dislocates dorsally relative to the metacarpal head. Clinically the MCP joint appears hyperextended. If the dislocation is complete, however, and the proximal phalanx and metacarpal are parallel, the extensive swelling can mask the deformity. The metacarpal head nonetheless is easily palpable in the palm.

Radiographic evaluation of MCP dislocations can be challenging (Fig. 8). In young children who have largely cartilaginous metacarpal heads, the joint simply may appear hyperextended on a lateral view. Alternatively an uncovered metacarpal head may appear prominently in the palm. On the posteroanterior view, the involved joint may appear widened or narrowed [19]. Radiographs should be inspected carefully for associated fractures, and oblique views are often helpful.

Dislocations of the MCP joint are anatomically different from proximal interphalangeal joint dislocations and frequently require operative

reduction. As the proximal phalanx migrates dorsally, the volar plate ruptures from its proximal insertion on the metacarpal and travels with the base of the proximal phalanx around the metacarpal head. The volar plate thus can become entrapped between the articular surfaces and can prevent closed reduction. Similarly the metacarpal head can become entrapped between the flexor tendons and lumbrical [20]. Attempts to reduce an MCP dislocation by longitudinal traction cannot overcome these forms of entrapment and may even transform a reducible dislocation into an irreducible type. Closed reduction attempts therefore should involve maintaining or exaggerating the hyperextension deformity while applying palmarly directed force to the base of the proximal phalanx. Infiltrating the joint with lidocaine or saline may help flush an entrapped volar plate out of the joint. If the dislocation cannot be reduced easily, operative reduction is required.

Open reduction commonly is required, especially in the index ray. The dislocated joint can

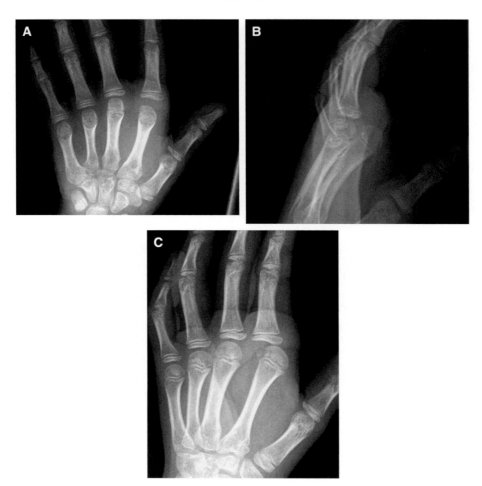

Fig. 8. (*A*) Anteroposterior radiograph of an irreducible index MCP joint dislocation. Note the widening of the index MCP joint. (*B*) Lateral view of the same injury. Note the uncovered metacarpal head protruding into the palm. (*C*) Oblique radiograph demonstrating not only the dorsal dislocation but also a displaced metacarpal head fracture not seen on the previous radiographs.

be approached volarly or dorsally. Proponents of a volar approach cite clear exposure of the incarcerating flexor tendons [17,20–23]. The digital nerves are tented over the metacarpal head, however, and are at considerable risk for injury during skin incision. In addition, the entrapped volar plate is displaced dorsal to the metacarpal head and is not well visualized through a volar approach, although the incision can be continued in a mid-axial direction to allow retraction of the volar plate from the joint with a skin hook [24].

Dorsal exposure of a dislocated MCP joint can be accomplished by retracting or splitting the extensor tendon. The dorsal approach has several advantages [8,25,26]. First, digital neurovascular structures are not at risk during the approach. Second, the entrapped volar plate is visualized easily dorsal to the metacarpal head. Reduction often can be achieved simply by incising the volar plate longitudinally and allowing it to reduce to either side of the metacarpal head. Care must be taken during the dorsal approach, however, not to inadvertently incise the flexor tendons, which can be draped dorsally over the metacarpal head and may be mistaken for the volar plate [8]. Finally, intra-articular metacarpal head fractures are easily evaluated and addressed through the dorsal approach after joint reduction has been performed.

After reduction of a finger MCP joint dislocation, the hand can be splinted or casted with the MCP joints in flexion for 1 week before initiating range of motion exercises. Concomitant fractures may require longer periods of immobilization. Redislocation or instability is uncommon in the finger rays. Patients and parents should be warned of possible untoward effects of these injuries, however, including osteonecrosis of the metacarpal head, growth arrest, deformity, and joint dysfunction [17].

## Discussion

Fractures and dislocations involving the finger metacarpals are common in children and adolescents. Not all fractures are treated easily and guaranteed a good outcome. The hand surgeon should be familiar with the variety of injuries in this region of the child's hand and should be able to evaluate and treat these injuries according to several key principles.

The location of the metacarpal fracture is important, within the bone and among the rays. Metacarpal base, shaft, neck, and head fractures behave differently and require different forms of treatment. Similarly, identical fractures in the index and small finger rays may require different treatment. Dislocations of the MCP and carpometacarpal joints are anatomically unique and pose distinct challenges.

The direction and location of displacement is as important as the degree of displacement. Rotational displacement is tolerated poorly and should not be accepted. Conversely in a young child many degrees of angular deformity in the plane of adjacent joint motion can be well tolerated and overcome by remodeling. The same degree of angulation at a metacarpal shaft is less well tolerated than at the metacarpal neck. Virtually any displacement of the metacarpal head articular surface should be reduced.

The mechanism of injury can give clues to associated soft tissue injuries that may be difficult to diagnose in young children. Crushing injuries, especially with multiple metacarpal fractures, should raise suspicion for compartment syndrome. Injuries sustained during a fight should be evaluated carefully for possible skin or tendon compromise.

Perhaps most important, not all principles of metacarpal fracture treatment in adults apply to children. Aside from the obvious remodeling potential and risk for growth disturbance in the growing hand, several differences between children and adults require underscoring. First, the periosteum surrounding the metacarpal shaft is thick in young children and can confer stability to many metacarpal shaft fractures that would be considered inherently unstable in adults and worthy of primary surgical treatment. Closed treatment therefore is more often successful in metacarpal shaft fractures in children than in adults. Second, children can heal fractures rapidly, especially in the metaphyseal regions. Although this speed of healing is helpful in most cases, it can allow a late-presenting fracture to progress rapidly to a malunion. Prompt treatment of displaced fractures therefore is required. Third, compliance with activity restriction and splint wear should not be relied on. If left to their own devices, most well-meaning but active children escape nearly any splint and play sports long before fracture healing. Casts are therefore preferable to splints when immobilization is truly important for maintenance of reduction or protection of pins. Finally, the supple joints of children are not plagued with the problems of stiffness that challenge the hand surgeon treating the adult patient. For instance, the MCP and interphalangeal joints can be immobilized in full extension for 4 weeks following a metacarpal neck fracture, and full range of motion typically is achieved within 1 to 2 weeks of cast removal with no formal therapy. In stark contrast to adults, early motion rarely is indicated in the setting of metacarpal fractures in children. With few exceptions (such as finger MCP dislocations and rigidly plated metacarpal shaft fractures), in children it is better to err on the side of too much rather than too little immobilization.

Despite the variety and potential complexity of metacarpal fractures and dislocations in children and adolescents, good results can be obtained with avoidance of common pitfalls and adherence to sound principles.

## References

[1] Hastings H II, Simmons BP. Hand fractures in children. A statistical analysis. Clin Orthop 1984;188: 120–30.

[2] Mahabir RC, Kazemi AR, Cannon WG, et al. Pediatric hand fractures: a review. Pediatr Emerg Care 2001;17(3):153–6.

[3] Rajesh A, Basu AK, Vaidhyanath R, et al. Hand fractures: a study of their site and type in childhood. Clin Radiol 2001;56(8):667–9.

[4] Valencia J, Leyva F, Gomez-Bajo GJ. Pediatric hand trauma. Clin Orthop Relat Res 2005;432: 77–86.

[5] Kleinman WB, Grantham SA. Multiple volar carpometacarpal joint dislocation. Case report of traumatic volar dislocation of the medial four carpometacarpal joint in a child and review of the literature. J Hand Surg [Am] 1978;3(4):377–82.

[6] Sandzen SC. Fracture of the fifth metacarpal resembling Bennett's fracture. Hand 1973;5(1):49–51.

[7] Whitson RO. Carpometacarpal dislocation; a case report. Clin Orthop 1955;6:189–95.

[8] Graham TJ, Hastings H 2nd. Fractures and dislocations in the child's hand. In: Gupta A, Kay SPJ, Scheker LR, editors. The growing hand: diagnosis and management of the upper extremity in children. London: Harcourt; 2000. p. 591–607.

[9] Graham TJ, Waters PM. Fractures and dislocations of the hand and carpus in children. In: Beaty JH, Kasser JR, editors. Rockwood and Wilkins' fractures in children. 5th ed. Philadelphia: Lippincott Williams & Wilkins; 2001. p. 271–379.

[10] O'Brien ET. Fractures of the hand and wrist region. In: Rockwood CA, Wilkins KE, King RE, editors. Fractures in children. Philadelphia: JB Lippincott; 1984. p. 229–99.

[11] Jahss SA. Fractures of the metacarpals: a new method of reduction and immobilization. J Bone Joint Surg [Am] 1938;20:178–86.

[12] Fischer MD, McElfresh EC. Physeal and periphyseal injuries of the hand. Patterns of injury and results of treatment. Hand Clin 1994;10(2): 287–301.

[13] Bogumill GP. A morphologic study of the relationship of collateral ligaments to growth plates in the digits. J Hand Surg [Am] 1983;8(1):74–9.

[14] Brown JE. Epiphyseal growth arrest in a fractured metacarpal. J Bone Joint Surg [Am] 1959;41-A(3): 494–6.

[15] Prosser AJ, Irvine GB. Epiphyseal fracture of the metacarpal head. Injury 1988;19(1):34–5.

[16] McElfresh EC, Dobyns JH. Intra-articular metacarpal head fractures. J Hand Surg [Am] 1983;8(4):383–93.

[17] Light TR, Ogden JA. Complex dislocation of the index metacarpophalangeal joint in children. J Pediatr Orthop 1988;8(3):300–5.

[18] Simmons BP, Lovallo JL. Hand and wrist injuries in children. Clin Sports Med 1988;7(3):495–512.

[19] Robins RH. Injuries of the metacarpophalangeal joints. Hand 1971;3(2):159–63.

[20] Kaplan EB. Dorsal dislocation of the metacarpophalangeal joint of the index finger. J Bone Joint Surg [Am] 1957;39-A(5):1081–6.

[21] Baldwin LW, Miller DL, Lockhart LD, et al. Metacarpophalangeal-joint dislocations of the fingers. J Bone Joint Surg [Am] 1967;49(8):1587–90.

[22] Cunningham DM, Schwarz G. Dorsal dislocation of the index metacarpophalangeal joint. Plast Reconstr Surg 1975;56(6):654–9.

[23] Green DP, Terry GC. Complex dislocation of the metacarpophalangeal joint. Correlative pathological anatomy. J Bone Joint Surg [Am] 1973;55(7):1480–6.

[24] McLaughlin HL. Complex "locked" dislocation of the metacarpophalangeal joints. J Trauma 1965; 5(6):683–8.

[25] Becton JL, Christian JD Jr, Goodwin HN, et al. A simplified technique for treating the complex dislocation of the index metacarpophalangeal joint. J Bone Joint Surg [Am] 1975;57(5):698–700.

[26] Bohart PG, Gelberman RH, Vandell RF, et al. Complex dislocations of the metacarpophalangeal joint. Clin Orthop Relat Res 1982;164:208–10.

ELSEVIER
SAUNDERS

Hand Clin 22 (2006) 11–18

HAND
CLINICS

# Fractures of the Phalanges and Interphalangeal Joints in Children

Anastasios Papadonikolakis, MD, Zhongyu Li, MD, PhD,
Beth P. Smith, PhD, L. Andrew Koman, MD*

*Department of Orthopaedic Surgery, Wake Forest University,
School of Medicine, Winston-Salem, NC 27157, USA*

Fractures of the metacarpals and phalanges of the hand are frequent. Hand injuries account for 2.6% of hospitalized pediatric orthopedic trauma [1]; fractures account for 19% of all pediatric hand injuries [2]. In a retrospective review of 354 pediatric fractures, hand fractures were common in the early teenage years [3]. A second and smaller peak incidence is seen in toddlers, related mostly to crush injuries in doors. Boys are injured more often than girls during sport activities or fights [2,4–6]. The rate of hand injuries during skateboarding, roller skating, and scooter riding is 5.8% [7].

Although 43% of injuries involve the proximal phalanx, the metacarpophalangeal joint is the most vulnerable site [4]; physeal fractures of the phalanges account for 37% of all physeal fractures [8]. The most common type is the Salter-Harris type II (54%) (Fig. 1). The little finger is involved most commonly (30%), and the thumb is involved in 20% of cases.

Most pediatric hand fractures can be treated by closed methods [9]. The time required for fracture healing in children is approximately half the time required for adults, and nonunion is rare. Immobilization for 3 to 4 weeks is sufficient for most phalangeal fractures in childhood; adolescents and teenagers often are treated identical to adults. Over treatment may be the source of complications [10]. In addition, children have a great potential of malalignment correction by

remodeling with growth [9]. Displaced fractures remodel in the plane of the joint remodel; however, rotational deformity does not correct. Unlike adults, sprains are uncommon in children and physeal injuries are more frequent than ligamentous tears.

In children poor outcomes often are related to delayed diagnosis secondary to non-recognition and late evaluation, inappropriate positioning during radiologic examination, and noncompliance. For these reasons the details of the injury are important to estimate the amount of associated damage or the degree of contamination with an open wound.

## Anatomic considerations

Knowledge of the anatomy and biomechanics of the normal hand is essential. The collateral ligament and dorsal and volar capsules are important and should be tested for stability before treatment. The collateral ligaments, originating from the collateral recesses of the phalangeal head, span the physis and insert on the metaphysis and epiphysis of the middle and distal phalanges. The accessory collateral ligaments insert on the volar plate. The collateral ligaments provide significant lateral stability and protect the physis, in part explaining the rarity of Salter-Harris type III injuries at the interphalangeal joints (Figs. 2 and 3). Forces directed laterally produce fractures on the proximal side of the joint rather than epiphyseal fractures [11].

At the metacarpophalangeal (MCP) joints of the fingers, the collateral ligaments originate from the metacarpal epiphysis and they insert on the

* Corresponding author.
*E-mail address:* lakoman@wfubmc.edu
(L.A. Koman).

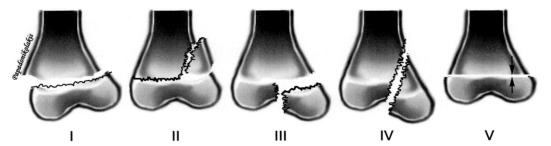

|  I  |  II  |  III  |  IV  |  V  |

Fig. 1. Classification of the epiphyseal plate fractures according to Salter-Harris. (Courtesy of Wake Forest University Orthopaedic Press, Winston Salem, NC.)

epiphysis of the proximal phalanx. Fibers originating on the distal metacarpal metaphysis represent an anatomic variation. The MCP collateral ligament inserts in two planes. This increases the frequency of Salter-Harris type III fractures at this level. The anatomy of the thumb MCP is similar to the proximal interphalangeal (PIP) joints. The volar plate is important in stabilizing the PIP and MCP joints and resists hyperextension forces. The volar plate inserts on the epiphysis of the distal segment.

## Diagnosis

### History and physical examination

The details of the injury are important to determine the amount of associated damage or

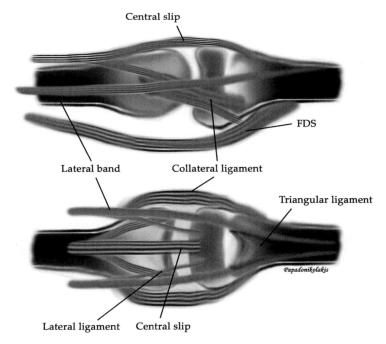

Fig. 2. The ligaments in the PIP joint reinforce the structure in three planes. The joint is stabilized on the coronal plane (adduction–abduction) from the collaterals that span the epiphysis and insert into the metaphysis of the middle phalanx. The insertion of the collaterals in the volar plate reinforces the joint in three planes—laterally, medially, and volarly—and decreases the risk for Salter-Harris type III fractures (top). On the dorsal site the joint is stabilized by the insertion of the lateral bands, lateral ligaments, and the central slip in the middle phalanx (bottom). (Courtesy of Wake Forest University Orthopaedic Press, Winston Salem, NC.)

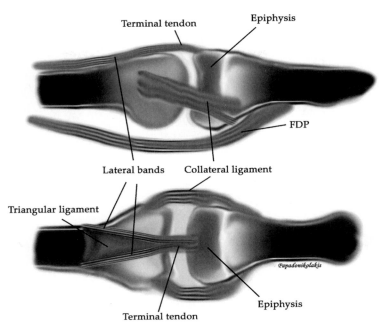

Fig. 3. In the DIP joint the collateral ligaments span the epiphyseal plate and insert into the metaphysis as in the PIP joint. Insertion in the volar plate provides stability in three planes and accounts for the rarity of Salter-Harris type III fractures at this level (*top*). On the dorsal site the joint is stabilized by the terminal tendon (*bottom*). (Courtesy of Wake Forest University Orthopaedic Press, Winston Salem, NC.)

the degree of contamination with an open wound. Children usually do not provide detailed information, thus the parents or caregivers should be asked about the mechanism of injury. Open wounds should be inspected carefully for foreign bodies and soft-tissue, nerve, or vessel injuries. During inspection, the posture of the hand may indicate specific bony or tendon injury. Edema, erythema, or bone/joint deformity should be noted. In children, physical examination is difficult to perform, because they are generally not cooperative, especially when they are in pain. If possible, assessment of the circulatory status, sensation, motor function, joint motion, and stability should be performed. The collateral ligaments and dorsal and volar capsules should be tested for instability before institution of treatment.

*Radiographic evaluation*

The radiographic assessment is important. Fractures should be evaluated in a minimum of two planes (posteroanterior, lateral) and oblique views are often helpful. Lateral radiographs are important to delineate rotation. Small fragments may be rotated on the attached collateral ligament

(Fig. 5) and may require open reduction and internal fixation [12].

**Treatment**

In general, closed reduction and immobilization with casting is recommended for Salter-Harris type I and II injuries (Fig. 1). The optimal position for casting is wrist extension and MCP flexion of 90°. Immobilization of the PIP joint for more than 3 weeks should be avoided if possible to prevent arthrofibrosis. Displaced Salter-Harris type III and IV fractures may require a closed or open reduction and osteosynthesis. Restoration of the joint congruity is important to avoid late osteoarthritis. The size of the fragment often determines the choice of fixation. For most of the Salter-Harris type V injuries, immobilization for 3 weeks is sufficient; growth arrest with loss of longitudinal development or angular deformity is not uncommon.

*Phalangeal fractures*

*Proximal phalanx*

Fractures of the base of the proximal phalanx (P1) are the most common pediatric hand injury;

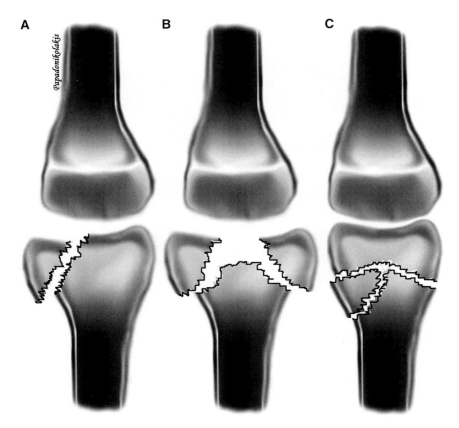

Fig. 4. (*A*) Unicondylar fracture of the phalangeal head of the first phalanx. Bicondylar fractures may have a Y (*B*) or a T (*C*) shape. (Courtesy of Wake Forest University Orthopaedic Press, Winston Salem, NC.)

most may be treated with closed reduction and splinting or casting. In a study of 37 children presenting with closed, unstable fractures of the proximal phalangeal head, active range of motion of the PIP joint after closed reduction was superior to open reduction [13]. Most P1 base fractures are extra-articular Salter-Harris type II physeal injuries (Fig. 6). The little finger is the most common site of injury (Fig. 7). Reduction is performed with the MCP joint flexed; it is

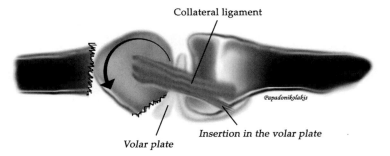

Fig. 5. Fracture of the head of the second metacarpal associated with rotation. The fragment may be rotated 180° and the articular surface may face the fracture site, rotating on the attached collateral ligament. The volar plate may be interposed between the distal phalanx and the bone fragment, making closed reduction difficult or impossible. Surgery is indicated to reduce the fracture. (Courtesy of Wake Forest University Orthopaedic Press, Winston Salem, NC.)

helpful to use a pencil as a lever for reduction. Once alignment and rotation are satisfactory, the finger is buddy-taped to the adjacent digit and a cast is applied with the wrist in 45° of extension and the MCP in 90° of flexion for 3 weeks. Radiographic review is suggested 3 to 7 days post-reduction to confirm that the fracture is not re-displaced. Entrapment of the flexor tendon within the fracture site may prevent reduction, necessitating open reduction [14]. Salter-Harris type III or IV fractures of the phalanges are usually seen in adolescents during the closure of the physis. Treatment should consist of K-wire fixation when the fragment has sufficient size. Stahl and Jupiter reported a technique of tension-band wiring consisting of placement of small-gauge wire through the insertion of the ligament into the fracture fragment [15]. The superiority of the technique lies in the reduced rate of complications compared with other methods of fixation. The fractures of the shaft of the phalanx are usually treated with immobilization along if there are stable [16]. Percutaneous pinning or screw fixation is often necessary, however, to avoid angulation or rotation deformities.

Condylar fractures of the head of the phalanx are classified by location and pattern as trans-condylar, unicondylar, or bicondylar. Transcondylar fracture lines are oblique and cross both condyles. Unicondylar fractures involve one condyle; and bicondylar fractures have a T or Y shape (Fig. 4). Minimally displaced head or neck fractures of the P1 frequently are missed; oblique radiographs are helpful in delineating the fracture patterns. Osteosynthesis often is indicated except in nondisplaced fractures.

The ulnar base of the proximal phalanx of the thumb may be fractured from forceful thumb radial deviation. The mechanism of injury is similar to an adult's gamekeeper thumb (ulnar collateral ligament [UCL] rupture). Ultrasound can be helpful in the diagnosis, especially in cooperative patients [17]. The conservative treatment with 3 weeks of immobilization is usually successful for minimally displaced fractures [18]. Open reduction and internal fixation is indicated for displaced fractures. Rarely the UCL avulsion may occur without a fracture [19]. Combined osseous and ligamentous injuries require the ligament and the bone to be repaired.

*Middle phalanx (P2)*

The treatment principles for the shaft fractures are similar to the P1 fractures. Fractures of the base of the P2 are usually Salter-Harris type III [20]. Most fractures are stable and 3 weeks of immobilization is sufficient treatment. Similarly to the palmar plate tears, adolescents may present with displaced volar fragments of the base of the P2. Open reduction is indicated when the displacement is more than 1 mm [21]. Salter-Harris type IV fractures are rare and can be associated with

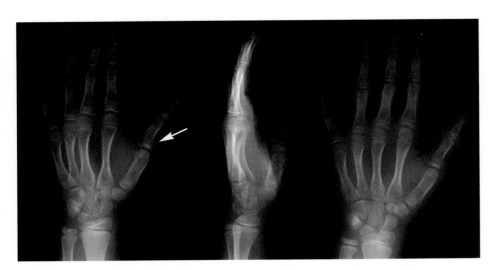

Fig. 6. These radiographs demonstrate the case of a 9-year-old child who had a fracture of the base of the proximal phalanx. The fracture line does not cross the articular surface, thus it is classified as Salter Harris type II. Notice the displacement in the lateral view (*middle*).

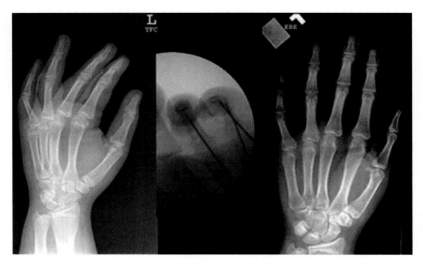

Fig. 7. These radiographs demonstrate fractures of the base of the proximal phalanges of the little and ring finger in a 13-year-old patient (*right*). Initially the fracture was treated with closed reduction and immobilization. The fractures were found to be unstable 5 days postreduction. Finally, pinning of the fractures (*middle*) resulted in healing of the fracture (*left*) with excellent range of motion and no cosmetic deformity.

poor prognosis because of the permanent damage to the growth plate.

The fractures of the head of the P2 may be associated with poor functional outcome. Almost half of them are associated with complications. Cartilaginous avulsion injury can be missed on initial radiographic study and is responsible for progressive stiffness or malrotation [10]. These fractures should always be treated surgically regardless of the degree of the displacement [21].

### Distal phalanx (P3)

Most P3 fractures are Salter-Harris type I or II. Splinting in neutral extension may be adequate with excellent or good results in most patients. Open fractures are common. They are usually associated with nail avulsion or laceration of the nail bed. Optimal treatment includes debridement, reconstruction of the nail bed, reduction of the distal phalanx, and pin fixation with K-wires. Reduction may be maintained with interfragmentary or transarticular pins. K-wires can be removed in the office in 3 weeks. The growth plate should be protected to avoid epiphysiodesis. The nail bed lacerations should be repaired under tourniquet control and loupe magnification after removing the nail plate [22].

The Seymour fracture is an extra-articular transverse fracture of the base of the P3 (Fig. 8). Before closure of the epiphysis, the fracture line is usually through the growth plate (Salter-Harris

type I or II) or 1 to 2 mm distal to the plate. It was first described by Seymour [23] and has received special attention because most often this fracture is open and often complicated with infection and premature physeal closure. Clinically these fractures mimic mallet deformities, although they do not involve the articular surface [24]. The deformity is caused by the different insertion sites of the terminal extensor tendon and the flexor digitorum profundus (FDP). The former inserts into the dorsal surface of P3 epiphysis, whereas the FDP spans the epiphysis and the metaphysis. The shaft of the distal phalanx is flexed by the FDP and the epiphysis remains extended because of the pulling of the extensor tendon. Although conservative treatment is usually successful [24], loss of reduction results in residual flexion deformity. Close follow-up with weekly lateral radiographs for the first 2 weeks of treatment is recommended to evaluate re-displacement. Al Qattan [25] recommended the use of a longitudinal K-wire fixation in noncompliant patients. Adequate debridement and the use of antibiotics for 5 days are important measures in avoiding infection.

In adolescents, avulsion fractures of the volar aspect of the distal interphalangeal (DIP) joint especially of the ring finger are common. In such cases an avulsion injury of the profundus tendon must always be suspected [26]. Sometimes these fractures consist of large bony fragments to allow K-wire fixation [26]. Pure avulsions of the

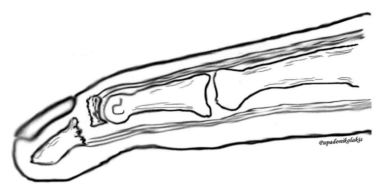

Fig. 8. The extra-articular transverse fracture of the base of the distal phalanx (Seymour fracture) is seen before closure of the epiphysis. The fracture line is usually through the growth plate (Salter-Harris type I or II) or 1 to 2 mm distal to the plate and mimics mallet deformity. The deformity is generated because of the different insertion sites of the terminal extensor tendon and the flexor digitorum profundus (FDP). The terminal extensor tendon inserts into the epiphysis of the dorsal surface, whereas the FDP spans the epiphysis and the metaphysis. The epiphysis remains extended because of the attachment of the extensor tendon. (Courtesy of Wake Forest University Orthopaedic Press, Winston Salem, NC.)

profundus tendon also may occur, requiring a direct tendon repair or a distal advancement with a pull-out button.

## Dislocations

### Distal interphalangeal and proximal interphalangeal joints

Although dislocations of the DIP and PIP joints are uncommon in children, dorsal dislocations are most frequent in DIP and PIP joints. Recommended treatment is conservative with closed reduction and progressive range of motion after 7 to 10 days of immobilization. Open surgery is indicated if the fracture is irreducible because of an interposed volar plate or unstable after reduction.

### Complications of phalangeal fractures

Malunited fractures cause cosmetic deformities and functional impairment. Rotational deformities result in overlapping of the fingers in flexion [12]. Early recognition of the degree and direction of displacement is important to avoid deformity. Malunited phalangeal fractures may be treated with osteotomy [27]. Partial or complete growth arrest may occur secondarily to the physeal injury. Avascular necrosis usually is associated with displaced unicondylar fracture caused by the disturbance of blood supply. Joint stiffness may develop as the result of malunion, arthrofibrosis, avascular necrosis, or infection. Dynamic splinting or physical therapy can be useful in the management of joint stiffness; however, younger children are not cooperative. In young children contracture may diminish with longitudinal growth. The status of the articular cartilage (articular stepoff of greater than 2 mm) and rotation are important considerations for surgery. Late capsular release and tenolysis are recommended rarely. Open fractures and fracture of the distal phalanges can be complicated by infection. Thorough debridement and appropriate antibiotic therapy are critical in avoiding infections. Salvage is difficult for arthritis and includes arthrodesis, interposition arthroplasty, allografts, and autografts.

## References

[1] Galano GJ, Vitale MA, Kessler MW, et al. The most frequent traumatic orthopaedic injuries from a national pediatric inpatient population. J Pediatr Orthop 2005;25(1):39–44.

[2] Bhende MS, Dandrea LA, Davis HW. Hand injuries in children presenting to a pediatric emergency department. Ann Emerg Med 1993;22(10):1519–23.

[3] Hastings H, Simmons BP. Hand fractures in children. A statistical analysis. Clin Orthop Rel Res 1984;188:120–30.

[4] Worlock PH, Stower MJ. The incidence and pattern of hand fractures in children. J Hand Surg [Br] 1986; 11(2):198–200.

[5] Blitzer CM, Johnson RJ, Ettlinger CF, et al. Downhill skiing injuries in children. Am J Sports Med 1984;12(2):142–7.

[6] Dohjima T, Sumi Y, Ohno T, et al. The dangers of snowboarding: a 9-year prospective comparison of

snowboarding and skiing injuries. Acta Orthop Scand 2001;72(6):657–60.

[7] Zalavras C, Nikolopoulou G, Essin D, et al. Pediatric fractures during skateboarding, roller skating, and scooter riding. Am J Sports Med 2005;33(4): 568–73.

[8] Peterson HA, Madhok R, Benson JT, et al. Physeal fractures: part 1. Epidemiology in Olmsted County, Minnesota, 1979–1988. J Pediatr Orthop 1994;14(4): 423–30.

[9] Salter RB, Harris WR. Injuries involving the epiphyseal plate. J Bone Joint Surg [Am] 1963;45:587–622.

[10] Wood VE. Fractures of the hand in children. Orthop Clin North Am 1976;7(3):527–42.

[11] Crick JC, Franco RS, Conners JJ. Fractures about the interphalangeal joints in children. J Orthop Trauma 1987;1(4):318–25.

[12] Dixon GL Jr, Moon NF. Rotational supracondylar fractures of the proximal phalanx in children. Clin Orthop Rel Res 1972;83:151–6.

[13] Bergeron L, Gagnon I, l'Ecuyer C, et al. Treatment outcomes of unstable proximal phalangeal head fractures of the finger in children. Ann Plast Surg 2005;54(1):28–32.

[14] Harryman DT, Jordan TF III. Physeal phalangeal fracture with flexor tendon entrapment. A case report and review of the literature. Clin Orthop Rel Res 1990;250:194–6.

[15] Stahl S, Jupiter JB. Salter-Harris type III and IV epiphyseal fractures in the hand treated with tension-band wiring. J Pediatr Orthop 1999;19(2): 233–5.

[16] Leonard MH, Dubravcik P. Management of fractured fingers in the child. Clin Orthop Rel Res 1970;73:160–8.

[17] O'Callaghan BI, Kohut G, Hoogewoud HM. Gamekeeper thumb: identification of the Stener lesion with US. Radiology 1994;192(2):477–80.

[18] Fischer MD, McElfresh EC. Physeal and periphyseal injuries of the hand. Patterns of injury and results of treatment. Hand Clin 1994;10(2): 287–301.

[19] White GM. Ligamentous avulsion of the ulnar collateral ligament of the thumb of a child. J Hand Surg [Am] 1986;11(5):669–72.

[20] McElfresh EC, Dobyns JH. Intra-articular metacarpal head fractures. J Hand Surg [Am] 1983;8(4): 383–93.

[21] Leclercq C, Korn W. Articular fractures of the fingers in children. Hand Clin 2000;16(4):523–34 [vii.].

[22] Zook EG, Guy RJ, Russell RC. A study of nail bed injuries: causes, treatment, and prognosis. J Hand Surg [Am] 1984;9(2):247–52.

[23] Seymour N. Juxta-epiphyseal fracture of the terminal phalanx of the finger. J Bone Joint Surg [Br] 1966;48:347–9.

[24] Ganayem M, Edelson G. Base of distal phalanx fracture in children: a mallet finger mimic. J Pediatr Orthop 2005;25(4):487–9.

[25] Al Qattan MM. Extra-articular transverse fractures of the base of the distal phalanx (Seymour's fracture) in children and adults. J Hand Surg [Br] 2001;26(3): 201–6.

[26] Leddy JP, Packer JW. Avulsion of the profundus tendon insertion in athletes. J Hand Surg [Am] 1977;2(1):66–9.

[27] Waters PM, Taylor BA, Kuo AY. Percutaneous reduction of incipient malunion of phalangeal neck fractures in children. J Hand Surg [Am] 2004;29(4): 707–11.

# Fractures and Dislocations Along the Pediatric Thumb Ray

## Scott H. Kozin, MD[a,b,*]

[a]*Orthopaedic Surgery, Temple University, Broad and Ontario Streets, Philadelphia, PA 19140, USA*
[b]*Shriners Hospitals for Children, 3551 North Broad Street, Philadelphia, PA 19140, USA*

The pediatric hand thumb is vulnerable to injury for several reasons. Young children inadvertently place their thumbs in vulnerable positions, such as doors and drawers. Adolescents participate in sporting recreational events, such as skiing, bike riding, or motorcycle riding, that require the thumb to participate in firm grasp. Skiing or biking mishaps frequently result in injury to the thumb [1–4]. In children, fractures and fracture–dislocations are more common than true dislocations, because the bone is more fragile than the ligaments.

## Relevant anatomy

The bony structure of the thumb is similar to a finger without a metacarpal. The physis is located at the proximal end of the distal phalanx, middle phalanx, and the metacarpal. This detail is important to remember, because the physis is most susceptible to fracture along the thumb ray. There are some normal bony variations that are worthy of mention. The pseudoepiphysis and double epiphysis are prime examples. A pseudoepiphysis is a persistent expression of the distal epiphysis of the thumb metacarpal [5]. The pseudoepiphysis does not contribute to growth, appears earlier than the proximal epiphysis, and fuses to the metacarpal by the sixth or seventh year. The prime clinical significance of a pseudoepiphysis is to differentiate this normal variant from an acute fracture. A double epiphysis is an active growth plate present on both ends of the metacarpal. The double epiphysis usually is seen in children with

a congenital difference. The presence of a double epiphysis does not affect the overall length of the thumb ray. Fractures can occur through a double epiphysis [5,6].

The insertion sites of tendons about the thumb influence fracture occurrence and deformation. The extensor pollicis longus tendon inserts on the epiphyses of the distal phalanx and the extensor pollicis brevis tendon inserts onto the epiphysis of the proximal phalanx. The abductor pollicis longus tendon has a broad-based insertion onto the epiphysis and metaphysis of the metacarpal. The abductor pollicis longus is the primary deforming force in most fracture–dislocations about the thumb carpometacarpal (CMC) joint [7]. The adductor pollicis inserts onto the proximal phalanx and into the extensor apparatus by way of the adductor aponeurosis. Epiphyseal fragments of the proximal phalanx with the attached ulnar collateral ligament (UCL) may be displaced outside the adductor aponeurosis. This pediatric Stener lesion prohibits healing and requires open reduction [8,9]. In contrast, the flexor tendons do not insert onto the epiphyses. The flexor pollicis longus and flexor pollicis brevis tendon inserts into the metadiaphyseal region of the distal and proximal phalanx, respectively.

The configuration of the collateral ligaments also influence fracture pattern. The collateral ligaments about the metacarpophalangeal (MCP) joints originate from the metacarpal epiphysis and insert almost entirely onto the epiphysis of the proximal phalanx. This attachment site explains the frequency of Salter-Harris (S-H) III injuries at the MCP joint level. The collateral ligaments about the interphalangeal joint are different. The collaterals originate from the phalangeal head,

* Shriners Hospitals for Children, 3551 North Broad Street, Philadelphia, PA 19140, USA.
*E-mail address:* skozin@shrinenet.org

cross the physis, and insert onto the metaphysis and epiphysis of the distal phalanges. Similar to the fingers, the collaterals also insert onto the volar plate to create a three-sided box that protects the physes and epiphyses of the interphalangeal joints [10]. This configuration explains the predilection of S-H II injuries at the thumb interphalangeal joint.

### Evaluation of pediatric thumb injuries

The evaluation of a child's injured thumb is more difficult than that of an adult, especially infants and toddlers. The child is frequently noncompliant, scared, and unable to understand instructions. Observation and play provides clues to the extent of injury. Fracture is evident by swelling, ecchymosis, deformity, or limited motion. Fracture rotation is detected by thumb position and comparison with the contralateral side. An older child can be comforted and relaxed, which allows palpation for areas of maximum tenderness. Stress testing about the MCP joint should be gentle to maintain the trust of the child. Sensibility testing is remarkably difficult in young children, because normal discriminatory sensibility cannot be tested until 7 to 9 years of age. A helpful examination to assess nerve integrity is the wrinkle test. Immersion of an innervated digit in warm water for 5 minutes usually results in wrinkling of the volar tuft skin. Wrinkling is usually absent in a denervated digit.

The clinical examination dictates the required radiographs. Areas of tenderness or ecchymosis warrant radiograph examination. Anteroposterior and lateral views are appropriate for screening. Oblique views may be added to further assess fracture configuration and displacement. Because the thumb is rotated 90° to the palm, anteroposterior and lateral radiographs of the thumb should be directed at the thumb and not the fingers. Placement of the palmar surface of the forearm and hand on a radiograph cassette and pronation of the wrist 15° to 35° with the thumb remaining in contact with the cassette provides a true lateral image [11].

The lack of ossification in the immature skeleton obscures bony detail and complicates radiograph interpretation. Indecisive interpretation requires comparison with the noninjured hand or consultation with a pediatric atlas of child development and normal radiographic variants [12,13]. The differential diagnosis of fracture is limited to nontraumatic entities that may resemble fracture (Table 1). A careful history and examination often exclude these diagnoses.

### Fractures of the thumb metacarpal base

*Mechanism of injury*

Thumb metacarpal fractures can occur from direct trauma, rotational forces, or axial loading

Table 1
Differential diagnosis of pediatric hand fractures

| Diagnosis | Characteristics |
| --- | --- |
| Trigger thumb | A trigger thumb can be confused with an interphalangeal joint dislocation because of the fixed flexion posture. The key diagnostic feature of a trigger thumb is the palpable nodule over the A1 pulley. |
| Thermal injury | Injury to the growing hand from frostbite, burns, or radiation may cause peculiar deformities from altered bone growth. In addition, thermal injury may lead to avascular necrosis of the physes or epiphyses. The end result is distorted bone width, length, or alignment that can be confused with fracture [14,15]. |
| Tumor | A tumor may be confused with fracture secondary to swelling or may be discovered after fracture through the weakened bone. An enchondroma of the proximal phalanx is the typical benign tumor that may fracture after trauma. Fortunately, malignant bone, cartilage, or muscle tumors are rare. |
| Inflammatory process | An inflammatory arthropathy (eg, juvenile rheumatoid arthritis, psoriatic arthritis, scleroderma, systemic lupus) may be confused with fracture secondary to decreased motion, swelling, and pain. |
| Infection | An infection is always in the differential diagnosis, especially in developing countries and immunocompromised hosts [16]. |

cause. Sporting endeavors are the principal activity leading to fracture.

*Fracture patterns*

In general, thumb metacarpal fractures can occur at the epiphysis (head), neck, shaft, or the base (Table 2). Fractures of the neck and shaft and their treatment principles are similar to those of the fingers (see articles on phalanges and metacarpal fractures by Papadonikolakis et al elsewhere in this issue). Thumb metacarpal base fractures are subdivided according to their location, involvement of the physis, and intra-articular extension (Table 2). These fractures are treated according to injury pattern.

Type A fractures occur between the physis and the junction of the proximal and middle thirds of the bone (Fig. 1). The fracture line usually is oriented in a transverse direction or slightly oblique to the shaft. The fracture often is angulated in an apex lateral direction, and medial impaction may be present.

Type B and C fractures are Salter-Harris II fractures at the thumb metacarpal base. The more common type has a metaphyseal fragment on the medial side (type B). In this case, the shaft fragment is adducted secondary to the adductor pollicis and pulled in a proximal direction by abductor pollicis longus. This pattern resembles a Bennett fracture with respect to the deforming forces, although there is no intra-articular extension [7]. Type C fractures are less common and have the metaphyseal fragment on the lateral side. The proximal metacarpal shaft is displaced in a medial direction. Type C fractures often result from substantial trauma and are not reducible by closed manipulation.

A type D fracture is a Salter-Harris III or IV fracture that involves the joint surface (Fig. 2). This type resembles most closely the adult Bennett fracture. The deforming forces are similar to an

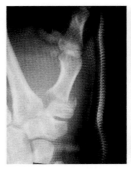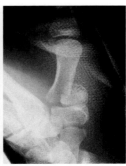

Fig. 1. A 13-year-old hockey player injured right thumb. AP and lateral radiographs reveal a type A fracture with considerable displacement. (Courtesy of Shriners Hospitals for Children, Philadelphia, PA; with permission.)

adult Bennett fracture and type B injury with subsequent adduction and proximal migration of the base–shaft fragment.

*Treatment*

The treatment plan must consider the location of the fracture and the status of the joint surface. Children have tremendous capacity to remodel extra-articular fractures, especially the thumb metacarpal. In addition, the extraordinary motion

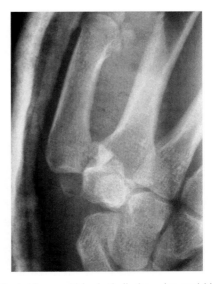

Fig. 2. A 14-year-old basketball player jammed his left thumb. Radiographs show a Salter-Harris III fracture of the thumb metacarpal base and an associated trapezium fracture. (Courtesy of Shriners Hospitals for Children, Philadelphia, PA; with permission.)

Table 2
Classification of thumb metacarpal fractures

| Location | Subtypes |
| --- | --- |
| Head | |
| Shaft | |
| Base | Distal to physis |
| | Salter-Harris II fractures—metaphyseal medial |
| | Salter-Harris II fractures—metaphyseal lateral |
| | Intra-articular Salter-Harris III or IV fractures |

at the CMC joint can compensate for mild persistent malalignment. For these reasons, extra-articular shaft fractures (type A) often can be treated by closed methods. In contrast, types B through D require physeal alignment and joint congruity to preserve growth and prevent arthritic changes.

*Type A*

Type A fractures usually are amenable to closed reduction and cast application. Swelling may delay closed reduction, because a brief period of cast immobilization (3–5 days) may be necessary to allow a diminution in swelling before closed reduction. Closed reduction requires longitudinal traction and pressure applied to the apex of the fracture to affect reduction. Residual angulation from 20° to 30° is acceptable, depending on the age of the child and clinical appearance of the thumb. The universal CMC joint motion and the potential for remodeling make this angulation acceptable. In addition, the fracture is located close to the physis and exact reduction is not required, because remodeling is plentiful [17,18].

Additional treatment is required in unusual circumstances. Closed reduction that cannot be maintained (unstable fractures) require closed reduction and pinning. Fractures that cannot be reduced (irreducible fractures) require open reduction and internal fixation (Fig. 3).

*Types B and C*

Simple closed reduction is more difficult for type B and C fractures. The mobility of the metacarpal base and the swelling make closed reduction more problematic. Treatment varies with the amount of displacement and degree of periosteal disruption. Mild angulation (<20°) can be treated by cast application without reduction.

Moderate angulation is treated with closed reduction and cast immobilization. Successful closed reduction requires short arm thumb spica splint or cast immobilization. Repeat radiograph evaluation should be obtained 5 to 7 days later to check the reduction [17]. Recurrent angulation requires repeat reduction and percutaneous pin fixation.

Severe angulation usually is combined with shaft displacement and warrants closed reduction followed by percutaneous pin fixation. If closed reduction is attainable but the reduction is unstable, percutaneous pinning is preferred. There are multiple options for pin configuration, including direct fixation across the fracture, pinning across the reduced CMC joint, or pinning between the first and second metacarpals.

An irreducible fracture requires open reduction and fixation. Comminution, soft tissue interposition, or transperiosteal buttonholing in type C fractures may prevent reduction [18]. Open reduction is performed to extricate the offending structure and pin fixation is performed to maintain alignment [18].

*Type D*

A type D fracture is a Salter-Harris III or IV fracture that involves the physis and the joint surface. Displaced Salter-Harris III and IV fractures are unstable and require closed or open treatment to restore physeal and articular alignment [19,20]. Closed reduction by way of longitudinal traction, adduction of the thumb metacarpal base (ie, abduction of the metacarpal head), and pronation of the thumb ray often attains fracture reduction. Direct pressure along the thumb metacarpal base may help push the shaft toward the avulsion fracture. The goal focus is to reduce the metacarpal subluxation and to restore articular congruity. Reduction is verified using mini-fluoroscopy and percutaneous fixation with two 0.45-inch (1.1-mm) trocar tipped Kirschner wires drilled through the thumb metacarpal and into the index metacarpal or carpus to hold the position. The Kirschner wires usually are left in a percutaneous position and protected beneath the cast.

Open reduction is required for irreducible fractures (Fig. 4). The preferred approach is volar, using a gently curved incision overlying the CMC joint along the glabrous border of the skin (Fig. 5). The cutaneous nerves are mobilized and

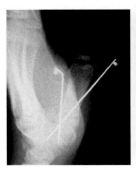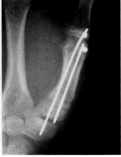

Fig. 3. Irreducible type A fracture depicted in Fig. 1 that required open reduction and Kirschner wire fixation to restore bony alignment. (Courtesy of Shriners Hospitals for Children, Philadelphia, PA; with permission.)

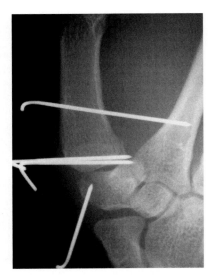

Fig. 4. Open reduction and Kirschner wire fixation was required to realign Salter-Harris III fracture of the thumb metacarpal base and associated trapezium fracture depicted in Fig. 2. (Courtesy of Shriners Hospitals for Children, Philadelphia, PA; with permission.)

protected. The attachments of the thenar eminence muscles along the metacarpal shaft are reflected. The CMC joint is isolated, opened, and exposed to reveal the articular surface (Fig. 6). Provisional reduction of the fracture is achieved under direct visualization. Subsequently, internal fixation is performed using Kirschner wires or mini-screws. Additional percutaneous Kirschner wire fixation between the first to second metacarpal often is performed to protect the fracture fixation.

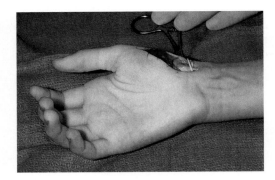

Fig. 5. Volar approach to CMC joint by way of curved incision overlying the CMC joint along the glabrous border of the skin. (Courtesy of Shriners Hospitals for Children, Philadelphia, PA; with permission.)

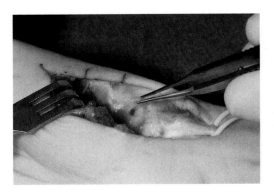

Fig. 6. The CMC joint is isolated by release of the thenar eminence muscles. (Courtesy of Shriners Hospitals for Children, Philadelphia, PA; with permission.)

## Postoperative care and rehabilitation

Closed treatment requires immobilization for 4 to 6 weeks, depending on the age of the child, fracture severity, and degree of soft tissue damage. After cast removal, a home program for range of motion is started. In active children and young athletes, a light splint may be used for protection for an additional few weeks. Formal therapy is rarely necessary, because a home program with instructions to the patient and parents regarding motion, strengthening, and activity return are usually adequate. The use of game systems is a common suggestion to promote thumb motion. Therapy may be necessary in complicated situations, such as considerable soft tissue injury or multiple traumas.

Early motion after rigid fracture fixation in children is controversial. The stability of the fixation and the reliability of the patient are important considerations. The physician must remember that fracture union with mild stiffness takes priority over fracture nonunion with excessive motion. A mature adolescent (who may be an oxymoron) can be allowed early-protected motion beginning 5 to 7 days after surgery. A removable splint is used for protection between exercise sessions until union between 4 to 6 weeks [21].

## Prognosis

Thumb metacarpal fractures often heal and thumb motion returns to near normal. There are numerous reasons for this outcome, including the remodeling capabilities of fractures near or involving the physis and the multiplanar CMC joint that is tolerant of slight malunion. In addition, residual deformity along the thumb metacarpal is better tolerated than the fingers, because digital scissoring is not a potential problem. Possible problems are physeal closure and joint incongruity (Fig. 7). Fortunately these complications are rare but do require early recognition and management to prevent long-term sequelae.

### Dorsal dislocation of the thumb ray

*Mechanism of injury*

Thumb MCP joint dislocations occur secondary to hyperextension. The thumb is especially vulnerable during sporting activities. The diagnosis is usually straightforward.

*Injury patterns*

Thumb dislocations are classified according to the relative position of the metacarpal and proximal phalanx, the integrity and position of the volar plate, and the status of the collateral ligaments. The classification is divided into incomplete dislocation, simple complete dislocation, and complex complete dislocation [22,23].

*Incomplete thumb metacarpophalangeal joint dislocations*

An incomplete dislocation is a rupture of the volar plate with partial disruption of the collateral ligaments. The proximal phalanx perches on the dorsum of the metacarpal. Closed reduction is attained by way of gentle longitudinal traction and MCP joint flexion. The limb is immobilized in a thumb spica cast for 3 weeks. Return to sports is delayed for an additional 3 weeks.

*Simple complete thumb metacarpophalangeal dislocation*

A simple complete dislocation is a rupture of the volar plate with complete disruption of the collateral ligaments. The proximal phalanx is displaced in a dorsal direction and is angulated 90° to the long axis of the thumb metacarpal. Closed reduction is more problematic, because excessive longitudinal traction may convert a reducible condition to an irreducible complex situation with volar plate interposition [24]. A successful reduction requires thumb spica immobilization for 3 to 4 weeks.

*Complex complete thumb metacarpophalangeal joint dislocation*

A complete or irreducible dislocation is the most severe type of dislocation (Fig. 8). The long axes of the proximal phalanx and the metacarpal are parallel and there is rupture of the volar plate and collateral ligaments. Open reduction usually is required to remove the volar plate from within the joint [22,23]. A dorsal or volar approach is appropriate; however, when using the volar approach, the physician must be wary of the close proximity of the neurovascular structures that are tented over the metacarpal head directly beneath the skin [24,25].

### Thumb ulnar collateral ligament injury at the metacarpophalangeal joint

*Mechanism of injury*

UCL ligament injuries are less prevalent in children than they are in adults. The pediatric injury is most common in the preadolescent or

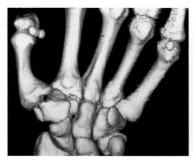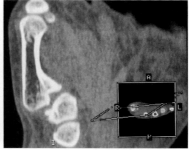

Fig. 7. A 21-year-old man with untreated Bennett fracture. CT scan and 3-D reconstruction reveal fracture malunion, articular incongruity, and joint subluxation. (Courtesy of Shriners Hospitals for Children, Philadelphia, PA; with permission.)

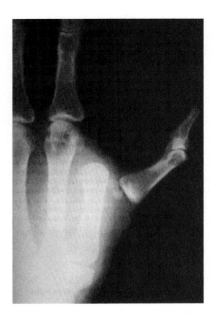

Fig. 8. Lateral radiograph of complete thumb metacarpophalangeal joint dislocation. (*From* Glickel SZ, Barron OA, Catalono LW III. Dislocations and ligament injuries in the digits. In: Green DP, Hotchkiss RN, Pederson WC, et al, editors. Green's operative hand surgery, 5th edition, volume 1. New York: Elsevier; 2005. p. 381; with permission.)

adolescent. A history of trauma is customary, especially sporting endeavors [26]. Skiing and extreme biking are specific activities that place the thumb MCP joint in a susceptible position. The mechanism of injury is a valgus or abduction force across the thumb MCP joint.

*Fracture patterns*

There are four types of injury patterns: (1) a simple sprain of the UCL, (2) a rupture or avulsion of the insertion or origin of the ligament, (3) an S-H I or II fracture of the proximal phalanx physis, or (4) an S-H III avulsion fracture of the epiphysis of the proximal phalanx that involves one fourth to one third of the articular surface [9,27]. In an S-H avulsion fracture, the ligament usually remains attached to the epiphyseal fracture fragment and may be displaced outside the adductor aponeurosis. This Stener lesion prohibits healing and requires open reduction to restore articular alignment and joint stability [8].

*Diagnosis*

The diagnosis requires a careful history and physical examination and warrants further discussion. A history of a sporting injury that places the thumb in jeopardy is an indication of UCL injury. The examination reveals swelling, tenderness, and ecchymosis about the thumb MCP joint. Tenderness often is well localized to the UCL and the pain is increased by abduction stress applied to the thumb MCP joint. A complete rupture or displaced fracture typically has more ecchymosis than a simple sprain. Most important, abduction stress lacks a discrete endpoint indicating complete UCL disruption or a displaced S-H fracture (Fig. 9). Anteroposterior and lateral radiographs are required. The radiographs are scrutinized for fracture and joint alignment (Fig. 10). Stress radiographs are performed only in ambiguous cases (Fig. 11) [26]. Advanced imaging studies (eg, MRI, ultrasound, and arthrogram) are always an option, although they should not supplant an astute physical examination and are not performed routinely in clinical practice.

*Treatment*

Simple sprains, incomplete tears, and nondisplaced fractures are treated by cast immobilization for 4 to 6 weeks. Complete ruptures or displaced fractures require surgery to evaluate for displacement of the ligament or fracture fragment outside the adductor aponeurosis (ie, Stener

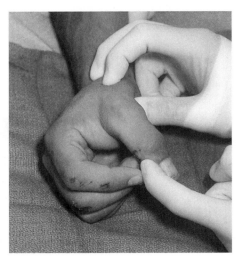

Fig. 9. A 13-year-old boy sustained a right thumb injury mountain biking. Valgus instability on stress testing without a discrete end-point. (Courtesy of Shriners Hospitals for Children, Philadelphia, PA; with permission.)

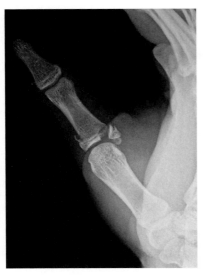

Fig. 10. Radiograph reveals a displaced Salter-Harris III fracture of the right thumb proximal phalanx. (Courtesy of Shriners Hospitals for Children, Philadelphia, PA; with permission.)

lesion), which prohibits healing [8,25]. An S-H III fracture that involves one fourth to one third of the articular surface of the epiphysis of the proximal phalanx is the most common pediatric pattern. A displaced fracture (displaced > 1.5 mm or

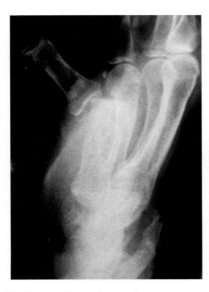

Fig. 11. Stress radiograph can demonstrate complete UCL injury and overt metacarpophalangeal joint instability. (Courtesy of Shriners Hospitals for Children, Philadelphia, PA; with permission.)

rotated fragment) requires open reduction and internal fixation to restore the integrity of the UCL and to obtain a congruous joint surface.

Surgical technique (S-H III fracture)

A gently curved incision is designed with curvature volar and ulnar to allow exposure of the volar fracture fragment. The skin is elevated with protection of superficial cutaneous nerves. The adductor aponeurosis, extensor pollicis longus, and extensor hood are exposed. A longitudinal incision is made along the attachment site of the adductor aponeurosis into the extensor pollicis longus (Fig. 12A). The underlying capsule is revealed and a longitudinal arthrotomy is performed. The joint surface is inspected and irrigated to remove any hemarthrosis.

The fracture fragment and joint surface is inspected and the type of fixation selected (Fig. 12B). There are multiple options, including Kirschner wire fixation, tension wire fixation, or mini-screw placement [26]. The author usually prefers tension wire fixation using a combination of a Kirschner wire and nonabsorbable suture [28]. The 0.045-inch Kirschner wire is drilled in an antegrade direction through the fracture site and into a percutaneous position along the radial side of the thumb (Fig. 12C). A second Kirschner wire is used to make an anteroposterior drill hole approximately 1 cm distal to the epiphysis. A small wire or nonabsorbable suture is placed through the drill hole, crossed, and passed through the UCL ligament at its attachment into the epiphysis (Fig. 12D). The fracture fragment is reduced and articular congruity is restored (Fig. 12E). The percutaneous Kirschner wire is drilled retrograde to capture the fracture fragment in its reduced position (Fig. 12F). The suture is tied in a figure-of-eight configuration to provide tension wire stability.

Closure requires careful repair of the adductor aponeurosis to the extensor pollicis longus. The adductor acts as a dynamic stabilizer to valgus stress and must be repaired. A thumb spica cast is applied that covers the percutaneous Kirschner wire. The thumb interphalangeal joint is not incorporated in the cast to promote gliding of the extensor mechanism. The Kirschner wire is removed 4 weeks after surgery and range of motion is started. A splint is fabricated to protect the repair during activities for an additional month. The splint is removed for exercises and activities of daily living.

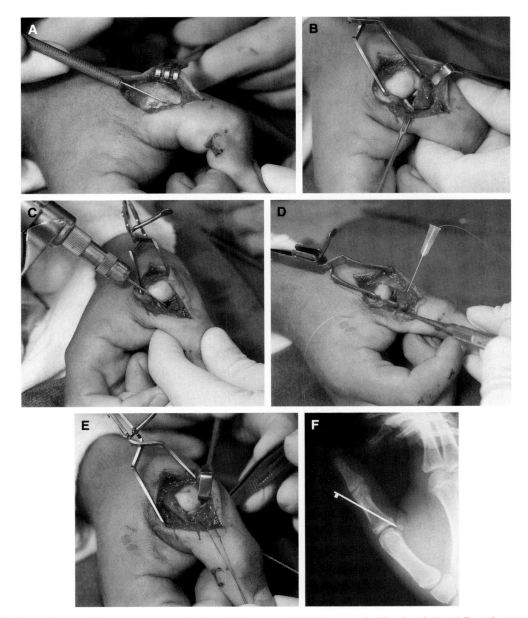

Fig. 12. A 13-year-old boy sustained a right thumb injury mountain biking, seen in Figs. 9 and 10. (*A*) Dorsal exposure and incision of adductor aponeurosis. (*B*) Arthrotomy and fracture exposure reveals an epiphyseal fragment that is rotated and displaced with UCL attached. (*C*) Antegrade Kirschner wire through fracture site and into a percutaneous position along the radial side of the thumb. (*D*) Thumb is rotated into pronation to expose the ulnar side of the proximal phalanx. Suture is passed through drill hole using a hypodermic needle as a guide. (*E*) Fracture reduced, percutaneous Kirschner wire advanced, and suture tied in a figure-of-eight fashion. (*F*) Radiograph after tendon band fixation with restoration of joint and fracture alignment. (Courtesy of Shriners Hospitals for Children, Philadelphia, PA; with permission.)

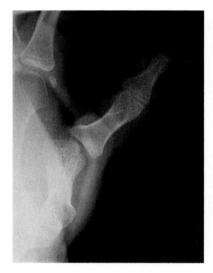

Fig. 13. An 18-year-old man with chronic UCL injury to right thumb after a motor vehicle accident resulting in spinal cord injury. (Courtesy of Shriners Hospitals for Children, Philadelphia, PA; with permission.)

Chronic pediatric UCL injuries are more difficult to manage (Fig. 13) [29]. Treatment variables include the time from original injury, age of the patient, level of impairment, and amount of MCP joint motion. UCL reconstruction is

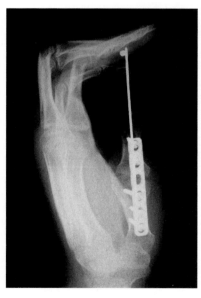

Fig. 14. Arthrodesis of the thumb metacarpophalangeal joint at the time of tendon transfers for tetraplegia reconstruction. (Courtesy of Shriners Hospitals for Children, Philadelphia, PA; with permission.)

complicated, especially in young children who have an open physis. Chondrodesis with an attempt to preserve the physis or arthrodesis has been the most reliable option (Fig. 14) [30].

## References

[1] Bhende MS, Dandrea LA, Davis HW. Hand injuries in children presenting to a pediatric emergency department. Ann Emerg Med 1993;22:1519–23.

[2] Hastings H Jr, Simmons BP. Hand fractures in children. A statistical analysis. Clin Orthop 1984;188: 120–30.

[3] Worlock PH, Stower MJ. The incidence and pattern of hand fractures in children. J Hand Surg [Br] 1986; 11:198–200.

[4] Worlock P, Stower M. Fracture patterns in Nottingham children. J Pediatr Orthop 1986;6:656–60.

[5] Haines RW. The pseudoepiphysis of the first metacarpal of man. J Anat 1974;117:145–58.

[6] Wood VE, Hannah JD, Stilson W. What happens to the double epiphysis in the hand? J Hand Surg [Am] 1994;19:353–60.

[7] Bennett EH. Fractures of the metacarpal bones. Dublin J Med Sci 1982;73:72–5.

[8] Stener B. Displacement of the ruptured ulnar collateral ligament of the MCP joint of the thumb. A clinical and anatomical study. J Bone Joint Surg [Br] 1962;44:869–79.

[9] White GM. Ligamentous avulsion of the ulnar collateral ligament of the thumb of a child. J Hand Surg [Am] 1986;11:669–72.

[10] Crick JC, Franco RS, Conners JJ. Fractures about the interphalangeal joints in children. J Orthop Trauma 1987;1:318–25.

[11] Billing L, Gedda KO. Roentgen examination of Bennett's fracture. Acta Radiol 1952;38:471–6.

[12] Greulich WW, Pyle SI. Radiographic atlas of skeletal development of the hand and wrist. 2nd edition. Stanford, CA: Stanford University Press; 1959.

[13] Stuart HC, Pyle SI, Cornoni J, et al. Onsets, completions, and spans of ossification in the 29 bone growth centers of the hand and wrist. Pediatrics 1962;29: 237–49.

[14] Hakstian RW. Cold-induced digital epiphyseal necrosis in childhood (symmetric focal ischemic necrosis). Can J Surg 1972;15:168–78.

[15] McCarthy JJ, Dormans JP, Kozin SH, et al. Musculoskeletal infections in children. Basic treatment and recent advancements. J Bone Joint Surg [Am] 2004; 86:850–63.

[16] Nakazato T, Ogino T. Epiphyseal destruction of children's hands after frostbite: a report of two cases. J Hand Surg [Am] 1986;11:289–92.

[17] Beatty E, Light TR, Belsole RJ, et al. Wrist and hand skeletal injuries in children. Hand Clin 1990;6: 723–38.

[18] Wood VE. Fractures of the hand in children. Orthop Clin North Am 1976;7:527–42.

[19] Gedda KO. Studies in Bennett's fracture: anatomy, roentgenology, and therapy. Acta Chir Scand 1954;5:193.

[20] Griffiths JC. Bennett's fracture in childhood. Br J Clin Pract 1966;20:582–3.

[21] Bergfeld JA, Weiker GG, Andrish JT, et al. Soft playing splint for protection of significant hand and wrist injuries in sports. Am J Sports Med 1982;10:293–6.

[22] Bohart PG, Gelberman RH, Vandell RF, et al. Complex dislocations of the metacarpophalangeal joint. Clin Orthop 1982;164:208–10.

[23] Weeks PM. Acute bone and joint injuries of the hand and wrist. A clinical guide to management. St. Louis: CV Mosby; 1981.

[24] Green DP, Terry GC. Complex dislocation of the metacarpophalangeal joint. Correlative pathological anatomy. J Bone Joint Surg [Am] 1973;55:1480–6.

[25] Stener B. Hyperextension injuries to the metacarpophalangeal joint of the thumb: rupture of ligaments, fracture of sesamoid bones, rupture of flexor pollicis brevis. An anatomical and clinical study. Acta Chir Scand 1963;125:275–93.

[26] Kozin SH, Bishop AT. Gamekeeper's thumb. Early diagnosis and treatment. Orthop Rev 1994;23:797–804.

[27] Mintzer CM, Waters PM. Late presentation of a ligamentous ulnar collateral ligament injury in a child. J Hand Surg [Am] 1994;19:1048–9.

[28] Kozin SH, Bishop AT. Tension wire fixation of avulsion fractures at the thumb metacarpophalangeal joint. J Hand Surg [Am] 1994;19:1027–31.

[29] Lipscomb PR, Janes JM. Twenty-year follow-up of an unreduced dislocation of the first metacarpophalangeal joint in a child. Report of a case. J Bone Joint Surg [Am] 1969;51:1216–8.

[30] Simmons BP, Stirrat CR. Treatment of traumatic arthritis in children. Hand Clin 1987;3:611–27.

ELSEVIER
SAUNDERS

Hand Clin 22 (2006) 31–41

HAND
CLINICS

# Scaphoid Fracture in Children

## Bassem T. Elhassan, MD, Alexander Y. Shin, MD

*Mayo Medical College, Department of Orthopaedic Surgery, Division of Hand Surgery, Mayo Clinic,*
*200 1st Street SW, Rochester, MN 55905, USA*

Carpal fractures are rare in the pediatric age group [1]. Scaphoid fractures are the most commonly fractured carpal bone with a peak incidence occurring between the ages of 12 and 15 years [2–8]. Scaphoid fractures account for 3% of all fractures of the hand and wrist and 0.45% of all fractures in the upper limb in children [6–9]. The low incidence of scaphoid fracture in children most likely is related to the thick peripheral cartilage that covers and protects the ossification center; as such considerable forces are required to cause scaphoid injury and fracture [10]. Because of the evolving changes in the ossification center of the scaphoid with age, the pattern of injury to this bone differs from that of adults [9,11,12]. During early stages of ossification, the scaphoid is more susceptible to soft tissue injuries and avulsion fractures, which explains why the most common pattern of scaphoid fracture in the child is the distal pole fracture [1,13]. The ossification progresses in a distal to proximal direction, and by early adolescence the fracture pattern becomes similar to adult types of scaphoid fractures.

The most common mechanism of injury is a fall onto the outstretched and pronated hand with tensile forces acting across the volar scaphoid [14]. Although the clinical presentation may not differ considerably from an injured adult, the relative rarity of this injury in children and the difficulty in interpreting radiographs of the immature carpus increase the rate of misdiagnosis [1,7]. This article reviews the development, mechanism of injury, associated injuries, diagnosis, classification, and treatment options of pediatric scaphoid fractures.

## Scaphoid development

The scaphoid is composed initially of articular cartilage, which covers extensive epiphyseal

cartilage that progressively undergoes enchondral ossification [3]. The cartilaginous model present in utero expands in size during prenatal and postnatal development. The ossific nucleus of the scaphoid appears at approximately 5 years and 10 months of age in boys and 4 years and 6 months of age in girls [15,16]. Multiple ossification centers occasionally may appear, but coalescence is rapid [17]. Enchondral ossification forms distally and grows in an eccentric mode until ossification is complete by the age of 15 years in boys and 13 years and 6 months in girls. The cartilaginous model of the scaphoid is completely ossified by skeletal maturity, and only articular cartilage covering most of the surface of the bone remains. The chondro-osseous transformation process depends on local perfusion supplied by a major vascular pattern of blood supply occupying the cartilage canal system throughout the postnatal development and maturation [6].

Malformation of the scaphoid manifested by bipartition was first reported after the work of Gruber and Pfitzner [18]. Gruber found four specimens among 3007 dissections and Pfitzner found nine examples in 1450 anatomic studies. They proposed that scaphoid bipartition is an infrequent developmental variation that results from failure of fusion of the proximal ulnar and distal radial components of the scaphoid [9]. They substantiated their work by demonstrating the notching at the ulnar side of the waist of the scaphoid as proof of incomplete fusion. Louis and colleagues believed that this condition does not exist and bipartite scaphoid essentially results from traumatic injury [18]. They performed dissection on 196 human fetuses with gestational age ranging from 4 to 30 weeks. Their dissections failed to identify any scaphoids with two equal and separate cartilaginous anlages. They also reviewed the hand radiographs of 11,280 children and were not able to demonstrate any case of bipartite scaphoid. As such, these investigators concluded that a bipartite scaphoid was a traumatically acquired condition resulting in asymptomatic pseudoarthrosis of the scaphoid.

## Mechanism of injury

The most common mechanism of injury is a fall on the outstretched and pronated hand [10,14]. In an older child, the mechanism of injury might be different. In a review of 64 cases of scaphoid fracture in children between the ages of 11 and 15 years, the most common mechanisms of injuries were sports in 27 patients, punching game machines or fighting in 22 patients, and traffic accident or other trauma in 15 patients [19]. The most common sports that yield scaphoid fractures in children are skateboarding and bicycling [1,13]. Minor trauma is the cause of scaphoid fracture associated with a pathologic process. This could be the first manifestation of a patient with scaphoid enchondroma [20]. In the nine cases with scaphoid enchondroma reported in the literature (eight boys and one girl), six of nine patients presented with fracture of the scaphoid after minor injury [21–25].

## Associated injuries

A more severe trauma is required to fracture the scaphoid in children younger than 10 years of age [17,26–28]. This is related to the thick cartilage that covers the bony ossification center in children, rendering the bone resilient, which necessitates considerable force to fracture the bone. The injuries associated with scaphoid fracture include supracondylar fracture [29,30], distal radius fracture [9,27,31,32], metacarpal fractures [17], capitate fracture (scaphocapitate syndrome) [33–36], other carpal fractures [3,37], and transcaphoid–perilunate dislocation [38,39]. The same mechanism of injury can cause concomitant failure of the bony and ligamentous structures in the arm, forearm, and hand. Despite the rarity of these associated injuries, careful clinical examination of the entire limb should be performed when a child has a suspected or diagnosed scaphoid fracture.

## Diagnosis

The clinical presentation of a child with scaphoid fracture may or may not differ from an injured adult, depending on the location of injury. The prevalence of distal pole fractures increases the likelihood of tenderness over the scaphoid tuberosity compared with the waist fracture with pain to palpation within the anatomic snuffbox. The relative rarity of this injury in children and the difficulty in interpreting the radiographs of the immature wrist increase the rate of misdiagnosis [1,7].

Swelling or tenderness over the scaphoid tuberosity or anatomic snuffbox or a painful scaphoid compression test (pain with axial loading of the first ray) should raise the suspicion of the presence of scaphoid fracture [40]. Posterior–anterior (PA), lateral, and oblique radiographs should be obtained. In addition, special scaphoid views consisting of anterior–posterior (AP) wrist views with bent fingers and with the wrist in 24° to 45° of supination can enhance visualization of the scaphoid. These radiographs place the scaphoid parallel to the film and reveal the scaphoid in its full size [41].

The physician interpreting the radiographs should be aware of the Pseudo-Terry Thomas Sign [42]. Because the scaphoid ossifies from distal to proximal, the distance between the ossified lunate and scaphoid decreases as the child approaches adolescence [42]. This leads to an increased distance between these two bones, with an average distance ranging from 9 mm in a 7-year-old child to 3 mm in a 15-year-old child. Failure to recognize these normal radiographic variants may lead to misinterpretation of a scapholunate dissociation, although in fact the apparent gap is filled with normal cartilage and unossified bone. Comparison with the contralateral wrist radiographs is extremely useful in distinguishing abnormal from normal patterns; however, one must keep in mind that carpal ossification is not always perfectly symmetric.

If the clinical picture is consistent with scaphoid fracture but the radiographs are negative, the patient should be splinted for 2 weeks and instructed to return for repeat examination and radiographs or magnetic resonance imaging (MRI) should be ordered. Many scaphoid fractures that are not visualized on the initial radiographs are diagnosed by way of MRI imaging abnormalities [43,44]. Fig. 1 shows the PA radiograph of a 12-year-old boy who complained of 3 weeks' history of right wrist pain that started after he fell on his outstretched right hand. His pain was localized primarily to the radial aspect of the wrist. He had mild swelling over the snuffbox area, which was tender to palpation, and a scaphoid compression test caused pain. Because the history and physical examination were consistent with scaphoid fracture, an MRI was obtained on his right wrist, which revealed a fracture through the waist of the scaphoid (Fig. 2A,B).

In a series of children evaluated with MRI, 56 children (57 injuries) underwent MRI within 10 days of injury [45]. All children had a suspected scaphoid injury but negative radiographs. In 33 (58%) of the 57 injuries, MRI was normal and the patients were discharged from care. In 16 cases (28%), a fractured scaphoid was diagnosed and appropriate treatment was initiated. Additionally, other fractures around the wrist joint and ganglion cysts were demonstrated on MRI. Despite the improved sensitivity of MRI in diagnosing scaphoid fractures in children, MRI does occasionally require sedation of the young child and may be overly sensitive, identifying bone edema as a fracture that never develops.

Bone scan [46], computerized tomography (CT scan) [47], and ultrasound [48,49] also have been shown to be effective in detecting carpal scaphoid injury. The role of bone scan has been nearly supplanted by MRI. CT scans are effective in the follow-up of scaphoid fractures to determine healing and are useful in determining scaphoid fracture displacement when operative intervention is indicated (Fig. 3). Ultrasound is used infrequently as a diagnostic tool for scaphoid fractures.

## Classification

Classification of the scaphoid fractures in children is based on their stage of ossification and

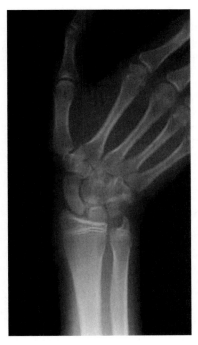

Fig. 1. PA radiograph of the right wrist of a 12-year-old boy shows no apparent fracture of the scaphoid. (Courtesy of Mayo Foundation, Rochester, MN.)

their radiographic features (Fig. 4) [50]. Type I fracture is a pure chondral injury involving children who are 8 years old or younger. As expected, because of its pure chondral nature, its diagnosis should be confirmed by MRI or one of the other advanced imaging modalities mentioned. Type II

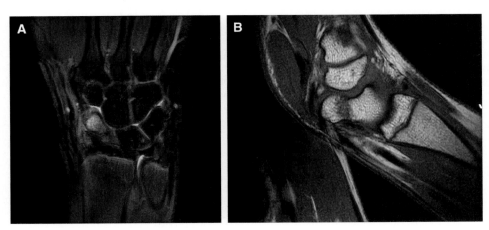

Fig. 2. (A) Coronal T2 weighted image of the right wrist shows a fracture through the waist of the scaphoid with bony edema. (B) Sagittal T1 weighted image of the wrist shows clearly the fracture of the scaphoid with minimal displacement. (Courtesy of Mayo Foundation, Rochester, MN.)

fracture is an osteochondral fracture that occurs in children between the ages of 8 and 11 years. Type III fracture occurs in children older than 12 years of age and transpires after the ossification center is well developed and the scaphoid bone is almost completely ossified. This is the most common type of scaphoid fracture in children. Each of these three types of scaphoid fracture may involve any part of the scaphoid, but it has been well reported that the most common pattern of injury involves the distal third of the bone, with tubercle fracture or avulsion considered the most frequent (Fig. 5A,B) [1]. This is related to the fact the scaphoid ossifies eccentrically with the distal pole ossifying before the proximal pole, rendering the distal-third fractures more common. The extensive cartilaginous structure of the immature scaphoid acts as a resilient protective cushion to the expanding ossification center, thus dampening the applied forces [51]. D'Arienzo reported on 39 scaphoid fractures in children. Most of the fractures occurred in boys aged 8 to 15 years, with more involvement of the right hand (27 of 39) [50]. Thirty-one fractures involved the distal third of the scaphoid, five fractures involved the scaphoid tubercle, and three fractures involved the waist. Thirty-one of these fractures were type III,

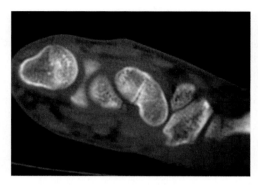

Fig. 3. CT scan of a 16-year-old boy with negative radiographs but persistent pain. Sagittal image reveals waist fracture without displacement. (Courtesy of Shriners Hospital for Children, Philadelphia, PA.)

six were type II, and only two were type I (purely chondral). In a similar study by Mussbichler [6], he analyzed scaphoid fractures in 100 children younger than 15 years of age and demonstrated that 52 fractures were avulsion of the radio-dorsal aspect of the distal end, 33 were in the distal third, and 15 involved the waist. In another study, Vahvanen [1] analyzed 108 fractures in children and found 49% of the fractures

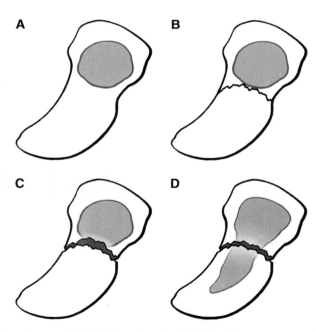

Fig. 4. Classification of immature scaphoid. (A) Normal scaphoid. (B) Type I fracture; a pure chondral injury. (C) Type II fracture; an osteochondral fracture. (D) Type III fracture. Adult variant fracture when the bone is almost completely ossified. (Courtesy of Mayo Foundation, Rochester, MN.)

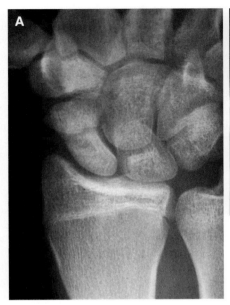

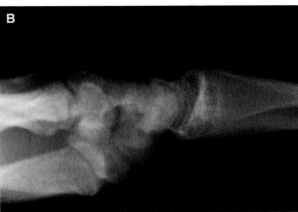

Fig. 5. (*A*) AP and (*B*) lateral radiographs of a 14-year-old boy who had a distal-third scaphoid fracture. (Courtesy of Shriners Hospital for Children, Philadelphia, PA.)

involved the distal third of the bone and 38% were avulsion fractures.

## Treatment

Any scaphoid fracture in a patient who has an open physeal growth plate of the distal radius and ulna is considered a pediatric scaphoid fracture. The younger the patient's age group, the more rare the incidence of scaphoid fracture. Only a few reported cases involve children younger than 8 years of age [1,15,17,52], and the youngest patient reported is 4 years of age [53].

Because of their great ability to heal and re-model, most of the scaphoid fractures in children can be treated with cast immobilization, especially because the distal pole is the most frequent location of scaphoid fracture in children (60%–85% in most series) (Fig. 6). In contrast with adults, the middle pole is involved less frequently (12%–38%) [1,6,9,15,27]. Proximal pole scaphoid fractures are rare, with only a few reports in the literature [28]. Most scaphoid fractures in children are also incomplete (disrupting only a single cortex) or are nondisplaced. Cast immobilization therefore is the gold standard of treatment of most pediatric nondisplaced or minimally displaced scaphoid fractures (Fig. 7A,B) [54–56].

For avulsion and incomplete fractures, a short thumb spica cast is recommended for 4 to 6 weeks.

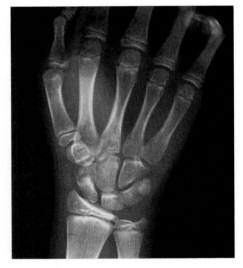

Fig. 6. A 12-year-old boy fell playing ice hockey and complained of right wrist and shoulder pain. Radiograph of right wrist reveals a distal-pole scaphoid fracture with slight comminution. Radiographs of the shoulder reveal a distal-third clavicle fracture. (Courtesy of Shriners Hospital for Children, Philadelphia, PA.)

In the younger child, a long arm cast may be appropriate to prevent the cast from falling off. For waist and transverse fractures, 6 to 8 weeks of immobilization is recommended. In the patient depicted in Fig. 1 who presented 3 weeks after injury and who was diagnosed by MRI (see Fig. 2A,B), treatment with a long thumb spica cast for 3 weeks followed by short thumb spica cast for another 3 weeks resulted in fracture union (Fig. 8).

In rare cases of proximal-third fractures, fractures that were neglected, or instances with apparent bony resorption, a longer period (8–12 weeks) of immobilization is recommended (Fig. 9). The immobilization begins with 6 weeks of long thumb spica cast followed by another 6 weeks of short thumb spica cast [1,27]. Fabre and De Boeck reviewed the literature and reported that of 371 children with acute scaphoid fracture treated with immobilization, only 3 (0.8%) developed a nonunion [13,57,58]. They found only 29 published cases of scaphoid nonunion in children. In their own series of 23 acute fractures of the scaphoid in children, all healed with cast immobilization. They also reported two cases of patients who had scaphoid nonunion who presented late after their injuries (referred from other institutions) at an average of 7 to 11 months after their injuries. Both were treated successfully with cast immobilization.

The blood supply of the scaphoid was described by Taleisnik [59], who suggested that the basic pattern does not change with growth. The retrograde, distally-based blood supply makes the risk for nonunion and avascular necrosis higher with more proximally located fractures. Because most pediatric scaphoid fractures are distal-third fractures, scaphoid nonunion is rare in children [60–67]. Factors contributing to nonunion are a delayed presentation or failure of initial diagnosis coupled with continued motion across the fracture site. Wilson-MacDonald recommended a trial of cast immobilization as the initial treatment in cases of delayed or nonunion of the scaphoid fracture [12].

Most scaphoid nonunions in skeletally immature patients involve the scaphoid waist (Fig. 10A–C) [65–67]. Mintzer reported a series of 13 scaphoid nonunions in children ages 9–15 years. The mechanism of injury in each case was a fall on the outstretched limb; nine of the 12 fractures occurred during a fall in a sporting event, and all fractures were waist fractures [68]. Preferred treatment and the average time elapsed between fracture and surgery was 16.7 months. All nonunions united after surgical stabilization.

A large series of scaphoid fractures (64 cases) contains 46 instances of nonunion [69]. The mechanisms of injury were mostly sports, fighting, and

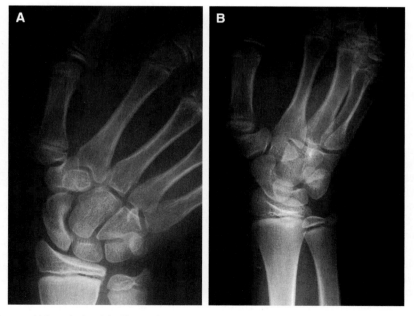

Fig. 7. The 12-year-old boy depicted in Fig. 6 after 8 weeks of casting. (*A*) Scaphoid view demonstrates healing of the fracture. (*B*) Pronated oblique radiograph further confirms fracture union. (Courtesy of Shriners Hospital for Children, Philadelphia, PA.)

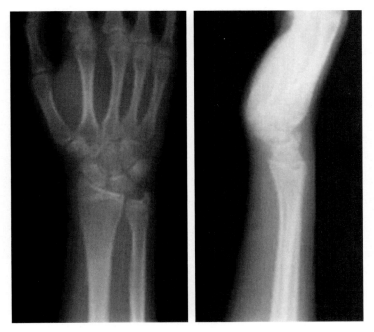

Fig. 8. AP and lateral radiographs of the right wrist of the patient depicted in Figs. 1 and 2 managed with 6 weeks of immobilization. Radiographs show a united scaphoid. (Courtesy of Mayo Foundation, Rochester, MN.)

punching game machines. All the nonunion cases were waist fractures except for one proximal and one distal pole fracture. The patients were between 11 and 15 years of age, and most injured presented late. There were multiple reasons for delayed presentation, including reluctance to tell their parents about their mechanism of injury, moderate symptoms that were not severe enough to seek medical attention, and fear of losing their position on a team.

There are multiple methods to manage a pediatric scaphoid nonunion. Union has been achieved by casting alone [70], casting with pulse electromagnetic field [62], Matti-Russe procedure [66,71], open reduction with bone grafting alone [67], bone grafting and Kirschner wire fixation [54], and open reduction with internal fixation using screw with or without bone grafting (Fig. 11) [65].

Mintzer and Waters reported their outcome in treating 13 scaphoid fracture nonunions in patients who had open physis of the distal radius and ulna [68]. The average time elapsed from time of fracture to time of surgery was 16.7 months. The average time for follow-up was 6.9 years. Four nonunions were treated by using the

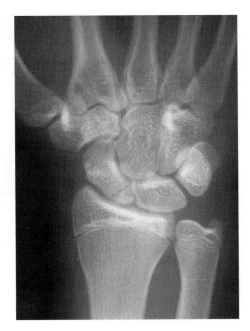

Fig. 9. AP radiograph of a 16-year-old hockey player (male) with a proximal-third scaphoid fracture. (Courtesy of Shriners Hospital for Children, Philadelphia, PA.)

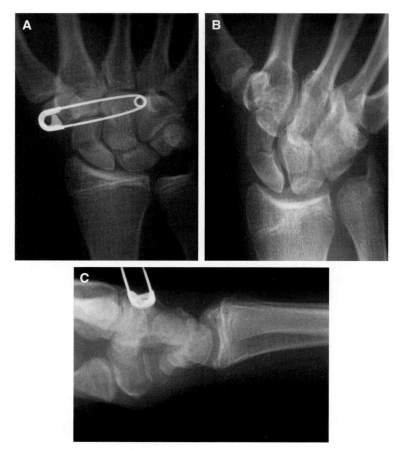

Fig. 10. A 13-year-old hockey player with persistent pain after diagnosis of wrist "sprain." (*A*) AP, (*B*) scaphoid, and (*C*) lateral radiographs demonstrate displaced scaphoid nonunion affecting the waist. (Courtesy of Shriners Hospital for Children, Philadelphia, PA.)

Matti-Russe procedure and nine were treated with Herbert screw fixation and iliac crest bone grafting. All the cases resulted in radiographic and clinical union. In all cases, the range of motion and strength between the operative and nonoperative wrist were statistically similar. The length of time for postoperative immobilization in the Herbert screw group was significantly less than that in the Matti-Russe group.

Toh and colleagues reported their experience managing 64 pediatric scaphoid fractures; 46 were nonunion [19]. The age of the patients ranged from 11 to15 years. The average time from injury to surgery was 74 days (range, 42–210 days) and the average time for follow-up was 27 months. Their indications for surgical intervention included acute (within 6 weeks) unstable fractures, fibrous union, and established pseudoarthrosis. Surgery

consisted of cannulated screw fixation in 52 cases, including 35 cases of bone graft. All cases except two achieved solid bony union (Fig. 12A,B). The functional results were not statistically significantly different between the acute cohort and the nonacute group. In the two nonunion cases, one patient was an ice hockey player who was noncompliant with immobilization. He required a secondary bone grafting to achieve bony union. The other patient was treated with open reduction and Herbert screw fixation and developed a persistent nonunion that necessitated repeat Herbert screw fixation and bone grafting to achieve bony union. This is the only patient who had decreased wrist range of motion and a diminished power grip compared with the nonaffected side.

No major complications have been reported from surgical intervention of scaphoid fractures in

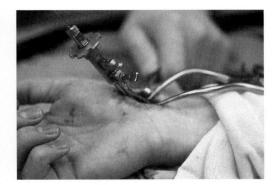

Fig. 11. Volar approach for bone grafting and screw fixation. (Courtesy of Shriners Hospital for Children, Philadelphia, PA.)

children. Concern has been raised, however, regarding the possibility of disturbing the normal growth of the scaphoid with the use of screw fixation [19]. Previous reports have suggested that smaller scaphoid screws may be preferred to accommodate the pediatric scaphoid and still provide rigid internal fixation [19,68]. In all the reported cases treated with screw fixation, the patients were 11 years or older. There is no report that explores the appropriate age that allows safe screw fixation.

Avascular necrosis of the proximal part of the scaphoid is possible but rare in the pediatric age group [3]. This is attributed to the prevalence of distal-pole fracture and that collateral circulation leading to restoration of blood supply may occur more readily in the child with resumption of the ossification process.

Scaphoid malunion resulting in humpback deformity is a known complication among adult patients who have displaced scaphoid fracture. Subsequently the lunate extends and a dorsal intercalated segmental instability results with limited wrist range of motion [72]. Correction of this deformity in adults involves osteotomy and bone grafting to restore the normal length of the scaphoid [73]. Because of the great ability of the bone to remodel in the pediatric age group, children are capable of remodeling a malunited scaphoid associated with correcting an intercalated instability pattern without the need for corrective osteotomy [74].

**Summary**

Scaphoid fractures in children are uncommon. A high index of suspicion is required in children when clinical signs and symptoms indicate a scaphoid fracture in a child. Radiographic evaluation with multiple views should be performed to

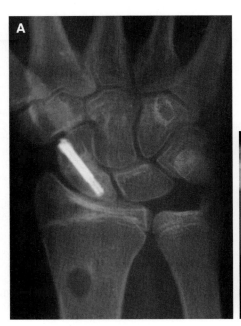

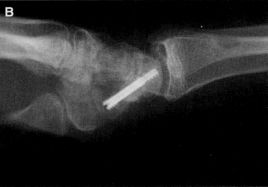

Fig. 12. (*A*) AP and (*B*) lateral radiographs after bone grafting and screw fixation with bony consolidation. (Courtesy of Shriners Hospital for Children, Philadelphia, PA.)

assess for fracture. If necessary, advanced imaging studies such as MRI should be performed. Most scaphoid fractures can be treated with cast immobilization, which results in healing in the vast majority of cases. Scaphoid nonunion is usually the result of delayed presentation or missed diagnosis. Fortunately union can be achieved reliably with cast immobilization or surgical fixation.

## References

[1] Vahvanen V, Westerlund M. Fracture of the carpal scaphoid in children: a clinical and roentgenological study of 108 cases. Acta Orthop Scand 1980;51: 909–13.

[2] Greene MH, Hadied AM, LaMont RL. Scaphoid fractures in children. J Hand Surg [Am] 1984;9: 536–41.

[3] Larson B, Light TR, Ogden JA. Fracture and ischemic necrosis of the immature scaphoid. J Hand Surg [Am] 1987;12:122–7.

[4] Light TR. Injury to the immature carpus. Hand Clin 1988;4:415–24.

[5] Mazet R, Hohl M. Fractures of the carpal navicular. Analysis of ninety-one cases and review of the literature. J Bone Joint Surg [Am] 1963;45:82–112.

[6] Mussbichler H. Injuries of the carpal scaphoid in children. Acta Radiol 1961;56:110–5.

[7] Nafie SA. Fractures of the carpal bones in children. Injury 1987;18:117–9.

[8] Kocher MS, Waters PM, Micheli LJ. Upper extremity injuries in the pediatric athlete. Sports Med 2000; 30:117–35.

[9] Christodoulou AG, Colton CL. Scaphoid fractures in children. J Pediatr Orthop 1986;6:37–9.

[10] D'Arienzo M. Scaphoid fractures in children. J Hand Surg [Br] 2002;27B(5):424–6.

[11] Cockshott WP. Distal avulsion fractures of the scaphoid. Br J Radiol 1980;53:1037–40.

[12] Wilson-Macdonald J. Delayed union of the distal scaphoid in children. J Hand Surg [Am] 1987;12:520–2.

[13] Stanciu C, Dumont A. Changing patterns of scaphoid fractures in adolescents. Can J Surg 1994;37: 214–6.

[14] Goddard N. Carpal fractures in children. Clin Orthop 2005;432:73–6.

[15] Wulff R, Schmidt T. Carpal fractures in children. J Pediatr Orthop 1998;18(4):462–5.

[16] Stuart HC, Pyle SI, Cornoni J, et al. Onsets, completions and spans of ossification in the 20 bone growth centers of the hand and wrist. Pediatrics 1962;29: 237–49.

[17] Bloem JJA. Fractures of the carpal scaphoid in a child aged 4. Arch Chir Neerl 1971;23:92–4.

[18] Louis DS, Calhoun TP, Garn SM, et al. Congenital bipartite scaphoid—fact or fiction? J Bone Joint Surg [Am] 1976;58:1108–11.

[19] Toh S, Miura H, Arai K, et al. Scaphoid fractures in children: problems and treatment. J Pediatr Orthop 2003;23(2):216–21.

[20] Takka S, Poyraz A. Enchondroma of the scaphoid bone. Arch Orthop Trauma Surg 2002;122: 369–70.

[21] Malizos KN, Getalis ID, Ioachim EE, et al. Pathologic fracture of the scaphoid due to enchondroma: treatment with vascularized bone grafting. Report of a case. J Hand Surg [Am] 1998;23:334–7.

[22] Masada K, Fujiwara K, Yoshikawa H, et al. Chondroma of the scaphoid. J Bone Joint Surg [Br] 1989; 71:705–8.

[23] Minkowitz B, Patel M, Minkowitz S. Scaphoid enchondroma. Orthop Rev 1992;21:1241–4.

[24] Redfern DRM, Forester AJ, Evans MS, et al. Enchondroma of the scaphoid. J Hand Surg [Br] 1997;22:235–6.

[25] Takigawa K. Chondromas of the bones of the hand: a review of 110 cases. J Bone Joint Surg [Am] 1971; 53:1591–600.

[26] DeCoster TA, Faherty S, Morris AL. Pediatric carpal fracture dislocation: case report. J Orthop Trauma 1994;8:76–8.

[27] Greene WB, Anderson WJ. Simultaneous fracture of the scaphoid and radius in a child. J Pediatr Orthop 1982;2:191–4.

[28] Pick RY, Segal D. Carpal scaphoid fracture and non-union in an eight-year-old child. J Bone Joint Surg [Am] 1982;12:441–3.

[29] Nashi M, Manjunath B, Banerjee RD, et al. Supracondylar fracture of the humerus with ipsilateral fracture of the scaphoid in a child. J Accid Emerg Med 1998;15(6):431.

[30] Stanitski CL, Micheli LS. Simultaneous ipsilateral fractures of the arm and forearm in children. Clin Orthop 1980;153:218–21.

[31] Sherwin JM, Nagel DA, Southwick WO. Bipartite carpal navicular and the diagnostic problem of bone partition: a case report. J Trauma 1967;11:440–3.

[32] Albert MC, Barre PS. A scaphoid fracture associated with a displaced distal radial fracture in child. Clin Orthop 1989;240:232–5.

[33] Sawant M, Miller J. Scaphocapitate syndrome in an adolescent. J Hand Surg [Am] 2000;25A:1096–9.

[34] Fenton RL. The naviculo-capitate fracture syndrome. J Bone Joint Surg [Am] 1956;38:681–4.

[35] Anderson WJ. Simultaneous fracture of the scaphoid and capitate in a child. J Hand Surg [Am] 1987;12A:271–3.

[36] Milliez PY, Dallaserra M, Thomine JM. An unusual variety of scapho-capitate syndrome. J Hand Surg [Br] 1993;18B:53–7.

[37] Kamano M, Fukushima K, Honda Y. Multiple carpal bone fractures in an eleven-year-old. J Orthop Trauma 1998;12(6):445–8.

[38] Compson JP. Trans-carpal injuries associated with distal radial fractures in children: a series of three cases. J Hand Surg [Br] 1992;17B:311–4.

[39] Hokan R, Bryce GM, Cobb NJ. Dislocation of scaphoid and fractured capitate in a child. Injury. Int J Care Inj 1993;24(7):496–7.

[40] Chen SC. The scaphoid compression test. J Hand Surg [Br] 1989;14B:323–5.

[41] Bohler E, Trojan E, Jahna H. The results of treatment of 734 fresh, simple fractures of the scaphoid. J Hand Surg Br 2003;28(4):219–331.

[42] Leicht P, Mikkelsen JB, Larsen CF. Scapholunate distance in children. Acta Radiol 1996;37:625–6.

[43] Cook PA, Kobus RJ, Wiand W. Scapholunate ligament disruption in a skeletally immature patient: a case report. J Hand Surg [Am] 1997;22:83–5.

[44] Cook PA, Yu JS, Wiand W. Suspected scaphoid fractures in skeletally immature patients: application of MRI. J Comput Assist Tomogr 1997;21:511–5.

[45] Johnson KJ, Haigh SF, Symonds KE. MRI in the management of scaphoid fractures in skeletally immature patients. Pediatr Radiol 2000;30:685–8.

[46] Waizenegger M, Wastie ML, Barton NJ, et al. Scintigraphy in the evaluation of the "clinical" scaphoid fracture. J Hand Surg [Br] 1994;19B:750–3.

[47] Bain GI, Bennett JD, Richards RS, et al. Longitudinal computed tomography of the scaphoid: a new technique. Skelet At Radiol 1995;24:271–3.

[48] Dias JJ, Hui ACW, Lamont AC. Real time ultrasonography in the assessment of movement at the site of a scaphoid fracture non-union. J Hand Surg [Br] 1994;19B:498–504.

[49] Senall JA, Failla JM, Bouffard A, et al. Ultrasound for the early diagnosis of clinically suspected scaphoid fracture. J Hand Surg [Am] 2004;29A(3): 400–5.

[50] D'Arienzo M. Scaphoid fractures in children. J Hand Surg [Br] 2002;27B(5):424–6.

[51] Grundy M. Fractures of the carpal scaphoid in children. A series of eight cases. Br J Surg 1969;56:523–4.

[52] Gamble JG, Simmons SC. Bilateral scaphoid fractures in a child. Clin Orthop 1982;162:125–8.

[53] Light TR. Carpal injuries in children. Hand Clin 2000;16(4):513–22.

[54] Maxted MJ, Owen R. Two cases of non-union of carpal scaphoid fractures in children. Injury 1982; 12:441–3.

[55] Ogden JA. Skeletal injury in the child. Philadelphia: Lea and Febiger; 1982. p. 363–4.

[56] Stewart MJ. Fracture of the carpal navicular (scaphoid). J Bone Joint Surg [Am] 1954;36:998–1006.

[57] Fabre O, De Boek H, Haentjens P. Fractures and nonunions of the carpal scaphoid in children. Acta Orthop Belg 2001;67(2):121–5.

[58] Langhoff O, Andersen JL. Consequences of late immobilization of scaphoid fractures. J Bone Joint Surg [Br] 1988;13B:77–9.

[59] Taleisnik J, Kelly PJ. The extraosseous and intraosseous blood supply of the scaphoid bone. J Bone Joint Surg [Am] 1966;48:1125–37.

[60] Barton NJ. Apparent and partial non-union of the scaphoid. J Hand Surg [Br] 1996;21:496–500.

[61] DeCoster TA, Faherty S, Morris AL. Case report. Pediatric carpal dislocation. J Orthop Trauma 1994; 8:76–8.

[62] Godley DR. Nonunited carpal scaphoid fracture in a child: treatment with pulsed electromagnetic field stimulation. Orthopedics 1997;20:718–9.

[63] Littlefield WG, Friedman RL, Urbaniak JR. Bilateral non-union of the carpal scaphoid in a child. A case report. J Bone Joint Surg [Am] 1995;77:124–6.

[64] Mintzer CM, Waters PM, Simmons BP. Nonunion of the scaphoid in children treated by Herbert screw fixation and bone grafting. A report of five cases. J Bone Joint Surg [Br] 1995;77:98–100.

[65] Onuba O, Ireland J. Two cases of nonunion of fractures of the scaphoid in children. Injury 1984;15: 109–12.

[66] Southcott R, Rosman MA. Nonunion of carpal scaphoid fractures in children. J Bone Joint Surg [Br] 1977;59:20–3.

[67] Caputo AE, Watson HK, Nissen C. Scaphoid nonunion in a child: a case report. J Hand Surg [Am] 1995;20:243–5.

[68] Mintzer CM, Water PM. Surgical treatment of pediatric scaphoid fracture nonunions. J Pediatr Orthop 1999;19:236–9.

[69] Horii E, Nakamura R, Watanabe K. Scaphoid fracture as a "puncher's fracture." J Orthop Trauma 1994;8:107–10.

[70] De Boeck H, Van Wellen P, Haentjens P. Nonunion of a carpal scaphoid fracture in a child. J Orthop Trauma 1991;5:370–2.

[71] Russe O. Fracture of the carpal navicular: diagnosis, nonoperative, and operative treatment. J Bone Joint Surg [Am] 1960;42:759–68.

[72] Nakamura R, Imaeda T, Miura T. Scaphoid malunion. J Bone Joint Surg [Br] 1991;73B:124–37.

[73] Amadio PC, Berquist TH, Smith DK, et al. Scaphoid malunion. J Hand Surg [Am] 1989;14A: 679–87.

[74] Suzuki K, Herbert TJ. Spontaneous correction of dorsal intercalated segment instability deformity with scaphoid malunion in the skeletally immature. J Hand Surg [Am] 1993;18:1012–5.

ELSEVIER
SAUNDERS

Hand Clin 22 (2006) 43–53

HAND
CLINICS

# Pediatric Distal Radius Fractures and Triangular Fibrocartilage Complex Injuries

Donald S. Bae, MD[a,b,*], Peter M. Waters, MD[a,c]

[a]Department of Orthopaedic Surgery, Harvard Medical School, 25 Shattuck Street, Boston, MA 02115, USA
[b]Department of Orthopaedic Surgery, Children's Hospital, 300 Longwood Avenue,
Hunnewell 2, Boston, MA 02115, USA
[c]Hand and Upper Extremity Program, Children's Hospital, 300 Longwood Avenue,
Hunnewell 2, Boston, MA 02115, USA

## Distal radius fractures

Distal radius fractures are among the most common pediatric injuries, comprising 20% to 35% of all childhood fractures [1–3]. Approximately one third of these fractures involve the distal radial physis [4]. Distal radial physeal fractures account for 25% to 50% of all physeal fractures, making them the most common growth plate injury of long bones, second in incidence only to physeal fractures of the phalanges [5–7]. With increases in sports participation among younger children, the incidence of forearm, wrist, and hand injuries has increased [8,9]. Furthermore, recent analyses suggest that increased body weight also may be contributing to increasing rates of pediatric forearm and wrist fractures [10,11].

### Anatomy

Developmentally, the primary ossification centers of the radius and ulna appear during the eighth week of gestation. The secondary ossification center of the distal radial epiphysis typically becomes radiographically apparent by the first year of life; rarely, there may be a separate secondary ossification center at the tip of the radial styloid. The distal ulnar epiphysis ossifies at approximately the age of 6 years in children and often develops from two distinct centers of secondary ossification. Knowledge of these patterns of epiphyseal development may assist in the distinction between subtle physeal injuries and developmental norms. Furthermore, comparison radiographs of the contralateral wrist may be helpful in these situations.

The distal radial physis contributes approximately 80% of the longitudinal growth of the radius. For this reason, fractures of the distal radius have tremendous remodeling potential. Indeed, previous studies have demonstrated that up to 10° per year of dorsal–volar angulation may remodel with continued skeletal growth [12–15]. Remodeling potential depends on several factors, including amount of growth remaining, distance of the injury from the adjacent physis, severity of angulation, and the direction of deformity. In general, younger patients who have fractures close to the physis in the plane of adjacent joint motion have the greatest remodeling potential. Rotational deformities have limited remodeling potential. Based on these principles, 20° to 25° of dorsal–volar angulation, 50% translational displacement, and 10° of radial–ulnar deviation may be expected to remodel with continued skeletal growth in younger patients [12–16]. These principles must be kept in mind when determining the optimal treatment for displaced distal radial fractures in skeletally immature patients.

### Clinical presentation

The diagnosis of distal radial fracture usually is not subtle. Patients typically present with pain,

---

* Corresponding author. Department of Orthopaedic Surgery, Children's Hospital, 300 Longwood Avenue, Hunnewell 2, Boston, MA 02115.
   *E-mail address:* donald.bae@childrens.harvard.edu (D.S. Bae).

swelling, or deformity of the affected wrist, typically after a fall onto the outstretched upper extremity. Careful evaluation of the skin should be performed to assess for a possible open fracture. A thorough neurovascular examination is performed similarly to assess for potential vascular or nerve injury or possible compartment syndrome. Plain radiographs confirm the diagnosis and serve to guide treatment. In general it is advised that the wrist and elbow joints are imaged appropriately to rule out ipsilateral injuries of the affected limb.

*Patterns of injury*

Distal radius fractures generally are categorized according to their anatomic location, pattern of injury, and degree of displacement, angulation, or rotation. These injuries may occur at the distal radius metaphysis or may involve the distal radius physis. Distal metaphyseal fractures generally are divided into torus or bicortical fractures.

*Management*

Torus, or buckle, fractures are characteristic injuries of childhood and commonly occur in the distal radial metaphysis owing to the increased porosity of metaphyseal bone, particularly during phases of accelerated skeletal growth. By definition, cortical failure occurs in compression, and as a result these injuries are inherently stable. Given their inherent stability, immobilization in a short arm cast or removable wrist splint for 3 weeks provides adequate symptomatic relief and prevents further injury. Recent randomized prospective studies have demonstrated that true torus fractures may be treated effectively and safely with splint immobilization and removed by parents after 3 weeks with no need for subsequent clinical or radiographic evaluation [17–20]. Typically there is little associated fracture displacement, and given the capacity for remodeling, fracture manipulation is not required.

Bicortical fractures of the distal radial metaphysis may occur because of bending, rotational, or shear forces sustained by the wrist during injury. These fractures may be transverse, oblique, or spiral in configuration and may present with significant displacement. Displaced fractures with unacceptable alignment may be treated with closed reduction and well-molded cast immobilization. The preference at the authors' institution is to use above-elbow casts.

The published recommendations of what constitutes acceptable alignment are highly variable, and there continues to be discussion and controversy regarding the indications for fracture manipulation and surgical treatment. In general, most authorities agree that up to 20° to 25° of angulation in the sagittal plane and translational displacement of up to 50% of the cortical diameter reliably remodel and may be accepted in patients who have greater than 2 years of remaining skeletal growth. In older patients, up to 10° of angulation in the sagittal plane and up to 10° of radioulnar deviation may be accepted.

It is important to recognize, however, that late displacement following initial fracture reduction occurs in approximately one third of cases. Inadequate reduction, poor casting techniques, resolution of soft-tissue swelling, muscle atrophy, and initial periosteal disruption all have been implicated as contributing factors to loss of reduction [21–23]. If the resultant deformity is deemed unacceptable or more than what may be expected to correct with fracture remodeling, further intervention is warranted.

Current indications for surgical treatment include irreducible or unstable fractures, open fractures, floating elbow injuries, neurovascular compromise, or soft-tissue swelling precluding circumferential cast immobilization [24–26]. Percutaneous smooth pin fixation may be performed following closed reduction to maintain appropriate fracture alignment. An oblique pin directed distal-to-proximal and radial-to-ulnar may be used, entering the radial metaphysis just proximal to the physis in an effort to avoid iatrogenic physeal injury (Fig. 1). A second dorsoulnar pin may be used to provide additional stability, though this is not always necessary if the affected limb is to be cast immobilized following percutaneous pinning. In instances in which appropriate percutaneous pin fixation cannot be achieved if an extra-physeal entry point is chosen, smooth pin fixation across the distal radial physis has been reported to be a successful treatment option with low risk for disruption of the distal radial physis [27].

Some investigators advocate percutaneous pin fixation for all displaced metaphyseal fractures in older children to avoid loss of reduction and need for re-manipulation. Pin fixation, however, carries the concomitant risks for infection, neurovascular injury, and general anesthesia. Randomized, prospective studies comparing the two treatment methods cite similar complication rates and no significant outcome differences [22,28].

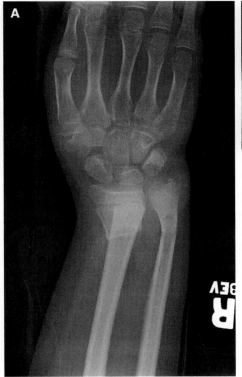
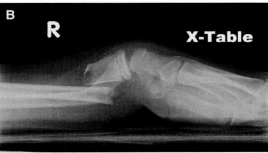

Fig. 1. (*A*) Anteroposterior (AP) and (*B*) lateral radiographs of the distal radius and ulna demonstrating a displaced metaphyseal fracture of both bones. This was treated initially with closed reduction and cast immobilization. There was subsequent loss of alignment and the patient subsequently underwent closed reduction and percutaneous pin fixation using a single smooth Kirschner wire entering proximal to the distal radial physis. (*C*) Postoperative AP and (*D*) lateral radiographs depicting appropriate pin placement, acceptable alignment, and bony healing (Courtesy of the Department of Orthopaedic Surgery, Children's Hospital, Boston, MA.)

Most distal radial physeal fractures are Salter-Harris type II fractures and are amenable to closed reduction and cast immobilization [29]. As with bicortical metaphyseal fractures, the authors' preference is to use above-elbow casts. Closed reduction should be performed atraumatically with adequate analgesia or anesthesia. Because of concerns regarding iatrogenic physeal injury, repeated reduction attempts or attempts at late reduction (greater than 5–7 days from injury) are discouraged. Indications for surgical treatment include significant soft-tissue swelling or concomitant neurovascular compromise (eg, compartment syndrome, acute carpal tunnel syndrome) precluding circumferential cast immobilization or intra-articular fractures with joint incongruity (eg, Salter-Harris III fractures) [26]. In these rare situations, percutaneous pin fixation may be performed using a smooth

Kirschner wire starting at the radial styloid and engaging the ulnar cortex proximal to the fracture site in a fashion similar to that described.

*Complications*

Distal radial growth arrest may occur following metaphyseal and physeal fractures. A recent study of 163 physeal fractures with average 25-year follow-up demonstrated a 4.4% rate of subsequent distal radial growth arrest. Distal ulnar physeal arrests were noted in 50% of cases [30]. In a similar study performed at the authors' institution, 290 skeletally immature patients treated for distal radial physeal fractures were studied in a prospective fashion. Overall, 4% of patients who sustained a displaced physeal fracture went on to demonstrate clinical or

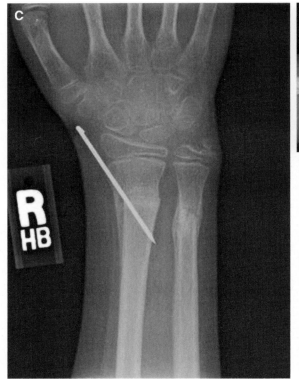

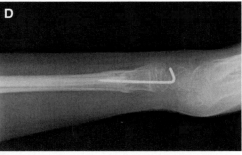

Fig. 1 (*continued*)

radiographic evidence of post-traumatic physeal arrest. Physeal arrest may be caused by the initial trauma and by iatrogenic injury. For this reason, late or repeated manipulations of displaced physeal fractures is not recommended, even in cases of severe deformity. Instead, observation with the expectation for remodeling is recommended. If there is incomplete correction of deformity with growth, a corrective osteotomy may be performed at skeletal maturity.

Patients who have displaced distal radial physeal fractures should be evaluated 1 to 2 years after injury to assess for possible growth disturbance. Significant radial growth arrest may lead to ulnar overgrowth and altered radial inclination, resulting in abnormal wrist mechanics, ulnocarpal impaction, possible triangular fibrocartilage complex (TFCC) tears, and distal radioulnar joint (DRUJ) instability. Depending on patient age, degree of deformity, and arrest pattern, physeal bar resection, radial osteotomy, ulnar epiphysiodesis, or ulnar shortening osteotomy may be

performed to improve function and prevent progressive deformity (Fig. 2) [31–35].

In a recent study from the authors' institution, 30 adolescents underwent surgical treatment for post-traumatic distal radial physeal arrest following previous physeal fractures [34]. Average age at the time of surgery was 14.8 years, and patients underwent distal ulnar epiphysiodesis, distal radial epiphysiodesis, ulnar shortening osteotomy, or corrective distal radial osteotomy, depending on the severity of the deformity and amount of skeletal growth remaining. Modified Mayo Wrist scores improved from 82 to 98 (maximum 100) in symptomatic patients following surgery, and ulnar variance improved from 4.5 mm positive to neutral in those patients undergoing ulnar shortening osteotomy. Preoperative symptoms and activity restrictions and functional limitations resolved postoperatively. Based on these results, the authors believe that surgery for post-traumatic distal radial growth arrest can improve pain and loss of motion in symptomatic

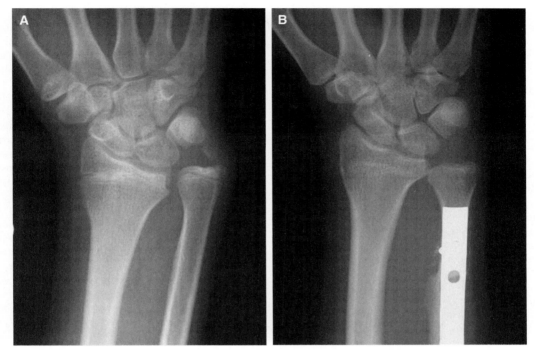

Fig. 2. (*A*) Preoperative AP radiograph of a patient who had post-traumatic distal radial physeal arrest and subsequent ulnar overgrowth. Note is made of positive ulnar variance and an ulnar styloid nonunion. Given persistent pain consistent with ulnocarpal impaction, this patient underwent ulnar shortening osteotomy, ulnar styloid nonunion excision, and open repair of the TFCC to the distal ulna. (*B*) Postoperative radiograph demonstrates restoration of neutral ulnar variance and a healing ulnar osteotomy site. (Courtesy of the Department of Orthopaedic Surgery, Children's Hospital, Boston, MA.)

adolescents and prevent symptoms in asymptomatic patients who have progressive deformity.

## Triangular fibrocartilage complex injuries

Though descriptions of TFCC injuries in adults have been widespread since the 1980s, only recently has there been increased understanding of similar injuries in the pediatric patient population [36,37]. Although this may be attributed to the increased awareness of these injuries, it is likely that increased sports participation in larger numbers of younger athletes also may be contributing to the increased prevalence [38,39]. Furthermore, as the use of diagnostic tools such as high resolution magnetic resonance imaging (MRI) becomes more widespread, so too may appreciation of the frequency of these injuries [40,41]. When present, TFCC injuries may be the source of ulnar-sided wrist pain in the child or adolescent. A thoughtful, organized clinical approach to these

patients allows for timely diagnosis, proper treatment, and return to activities.

### Anatomy

The TFCC refers to a convergence of structures on the ulnar side of the wrist that serve to support the ulnocarpal articulation and stabilize the DRUJ. First described by Palmer and Werner, these structures include the triangular fibrocartilage, the dorsal and volar radioulnar ligaments, the meniscal homolog, the ulnolunate and ulnotriquetral ligaments, and the subsheath of the extensor carpi ulnaris (ECU) tendon [36]. Functionally the TFCC provides a smooth articular surface between the radius and ulna, transmits and absorbs axial loads across the ulnocarpal articulation, and contributes stability to the ulnar wrist and DRUJ. Previous studies have demonstrated that approximately 20% of the axial load is transmitted across the ulnocarpal joint in wrists with neutral ulnar variance [42]. Small changes in ulnar variance may result in significant alterations in axial loads borne by the TFCC.

## Clinical presentation

Most patients who have TFCC tears present with ulnar-sided wrist pain, typically exacerbated with forceful grip and twisting-type activities. Often there has been a history of antecedent wrist trauma, and it is believed that most TFCC injuries arise from axially loading of or fall onto the extended and pronated wrist [43]. Many patients have had treatment for prior distal radius or ulna fractures. It is important to recognize, however, that the symptoms of TFCC injury may be subtle, particularly in the child or adolescent. Indeed, patients may complain of wrist pain only during specific sports-related activity and may be free of pain or functional limitations during activities of daily living [37].

Physical examination findings also may be subtle. Usually there is tenderness over the ulnar aspect of the wrist. The TFCC compression test, in which the wrist is axially loaded, ulnarly deviated, and rotated, is a helpful provocative test. Similarly the integrity of the DRUJ must be assessed, because TFCC disruption may be associated with DRUJ instability.

All patients who have suspected TFCC injury should be evaluated with plain radiographs. Radiographs are performed to identify potential coexisting wrist pathology, including distal radial fracture malunion, ulnar styloid nonunion, positive ulnar variance with ulnocarpal impaction, and DRUJ instability. As the apparent length of the distal ulna can vary with forearm rotation, standardized views should be obtained and variance measured according to the technique of perpendiculars [44]. Comparison radiographs of the contralateral wrist may be useful in these situations.

MRI may be used to assess the integrity of the TFCC. Though early reports of this imaging modality noted significant limitations in the evaluation of the TFCC, the sensitivity and specificity of MRI has improved [40,41,45]. Patients who have persistent pain and functional limitations associated with TFCC injury despite rest, activity modification, and physical/occupational therapy are candidates for surgical treatment.

## Patterns of injury

The Palmer classification is the system used most commonly to describe TFCC injuries [46]. In the pediatric population, traumatic (class 1) injuries represent the vast majority of TFCC tears; as expected, degenerative (class 2) tears of the TFCC are far less common. Injuries to the TFCC are further classified based on the location of the cartilage complex tear (Table 1).

Based on previously published reports, there is an apparent increased prevalence of Palmer 1B tears in pediatric patients compared with adults [37,47]. Indeed, the authors believe these tears from the ulnar attachment—with or without associated ulnar styloid fractures—represent the most common variety of TFCC injuries in children and adolescents.

Tears of the radial attachment (Palmer 1D tears) represent the second most common type of TFCC injuries in children and adolescents. Great care should be taken during preoperative evaluation, MRI analysis, and intraoperative arthroscopic survey to ensure accurate diagnosis of these radial-sided tears. If mistaken for a central traumatic tear (Palmer 1A), simple debridement alone in these situations may result in persistent pain, instability, and functional limitations.

## Surgical management

In appropriate patients who have peripheral TFCC tears, the authors currently advocate arthroscopically-assisted suture repair of the TFCC to its ulnar or radial attachments. Diagnostic wrist arthroscopy is performed in the

Table 1
Classification of TFCC tears

| | |
|---|---|
| **Class 1: traumatic** | |
| A | Central perforation |
| B | Ulnar avulsion |
| C | Distal avulsion |
| D | Radial avulsion |
| **Class 2: degenerative** | |
| A | TFCC wear |
| B | TFCC wear, lunate/ulnar chondromalacia |
| C | TFCC perforation, lunate/ulnar chondromalacia |
| D | TFCC perforation, lunate/ulnar chondromalacia, LT ligament perforation |
| E | TFCC perforation, lunate/ulnar chondromalacia, LT ligament perforation, ulnocarpal arthritis |

*From* Palmer AK. Triangular fibrocastilage complex lesions: a classification. J Hand Surg [Am] 1989;14: 594–606; with permission.

usual fashion, with the arthroscope placed in the 3-4 portal [48]. The 4-5 or 6R portal typically is used as the working portal. Debridement of the edge of the TFCC tear and adjacent synovium is performed using a size-appropriate arthroscopic shaver; a bleeding surface thus is created at the planned repair site to promote soft tissue healing.

In cases of Palmer 1B tears, the authors advocate an outside-in technique using Tuohy needles or commercially available suture passers (Fig. 3) [49,50]. Using an outside-in technique, 18-gauge Tuohy needles are inserted percutaneously on the ulnar side of the wrist, with care being taken to stay dorsal to the flexor carpi ulnaris

tendon in an effort to avoid neurovascular embarrassment/compromise [51–53]. These needles are passed into the site of the tear, brought through the undersurface of the TFCC, and subsequently used to pierce the ulnar margin of the intact fibrocartilage. Number 2-0 polydioxanone sutures are passed down one needle across the TFCC and shuttled out the adjacent Tuohy needle, completing a horizontal mattress stitch. A small incision is created in the skin at the site of suture entry, and careful subcutaneous spreading is performed to ensure that branches of the dorsoulnar sensory nerve are not entrapped in the suture strands. The suture then is tensioned and tied over the wrist

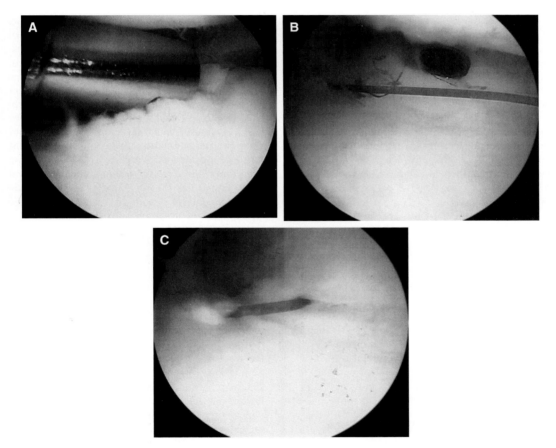

Fig. 3. Arthroscopic-assisted repair of a peripheral Palmer 1B TFCC tear in the left wrist. (*A*) With the arthroscope in 3-4 portal, visualization is made of the ulnar-sided TFCC tear. The proximal edge of the triquetrum is seen in the superior portion of the field. A small full-radius shaver has been introduced by way of the 4-5 portal and debridement of the tear and adjacent synovium is performed. (*B*) Tuohy needles introduced percutaneously from the ulnar side of the wrist are passed through the site of the tear and the intact ulnar edge of the triangular fibrocartilage. A 2-0 polydioxanone is passed through these needles to facilitate repair. (*C*) As the suture is tensioned and tied over the ulnar wrist capsule with care being taken to avoid iatrogenic injury to the dorsal sensory branch of the ulnar nerve, the TFCC repair is completed. (Courtesy of the Department of Orthopaedic Surgery, Children's Hospital, Boston, MA.)

capsule, reapproximating the TFCC to its ulnar insertion and completing a horizontal mattress repair. It is advisable to remove the operative extremity from traction and position the wrist in neutral rotation and slight ulnar deviation before tying down the suture. Although the authors currently use the outside-in technique of TFCC repair, inside-out, open, and all arthroscopic methods have been used by other investigators with similar success [54,55].

The same surgical principles are followed during arthroscopically-assisted repair of Palmer type ID lesions, with slight technical modifications [47,52]. Following wrist arthroscopy and synovial debridement, the radial attachment of the TFCC is identified. A 2-0 polydioxanone suture with each end loaded onto long straight needles then is passed from the ulnar border of the wrist. Long Keith needles also may be used for this purpose. The needles are passed through the intact radial TFCC, brought into the tear, and subsequently passed directly through the radius, exiting between the first and second dorsal extensor compartments. The long straight needles may be drilled through the radial metaphysis or passed through previously placed channels created by percutaneous Kirschner wires. The horizontal mattress repair then is completed by tensioning the TFCC and tying the sutures over the distal radial metaphysis.

Postoperatively, patients are immobilized in long-arm casts with the elbow flexed 90° and the forearm in supination for 4 weeks, followed by short-arm casts or splints for an additional 2 weeks. Range of motion and strengthening exercises then are initiated. Sports participation is allowed after 3 months.

It is imperative that coexisting wrist pathology be addressed at the time of surgical treatment. Failure to do so may result in recurrent TFCC tears, persistent pain, and suboptimal outcomes. In particular, special care should be taken to address associated ulnar styloid nonunions, ulnocarpal impaction in the setting of positive ulnar variance, and DRUJ instability. Fractures through the base of the ulnar styloid may be associated with TFCC disruption and DRUJ instability, because the TFCC remains attached to the displaced fracture fragment. In general, ununited ulnar styloid fractures may be treated by fracture fixation or styloid excision [56,57]. Open reduction and internal fixation typically is performed by way of a direct ulnar approach to the distal ulna, with care being taken to protect the sensory branches of the ulnar nerve. After the fracture has been exposed, debrided, and anatomically reduced, fixation may be performed using compression screw or tension band technique. Care should be made to ensure that DRUJ congruity and stability have been achieved on completion of the ulnar styloid repair. Excision of the ulnar styloid with subsequent repair of the TFCC to the distal ulna is also effective. In these situations, the distal ulna typically is approached dorsally between the fifth and sixth extensor compartments. After styloid excision, the distal ulna is debrided back to bleeding bone and the ulnar border of the TFCC is repaired using sutures passed through drill holes. Again, DRUJ stability is confirmed following TFCC repair. Although wafer distal ulna resection has been advocated by some investigators in adults for the treatment of TFCC tears in the setting of positive ulnar variance, these techniques rely on the presence of a central, degenerative TFCC tear (Palmer type II) and mechanical debridement of the distal ulnar articular surface [58]. The authors do not advocate the use of wafer distal ulna resection for TFCC tears or ulnocarpal impaction in the pediatric patient population. Instead, positive ulnar variance is addressed with open ulnar shortening osteotomy, fixed with compression plate and screw constructs [59,60]. Finally, in those cases in which DRUJ instability persists after the TFCC tears or ulnar styloid fractures have been appropriately addressed, reinforcement of the DRUJ ligament or formal ligament reconstruction may be performed.

*Results of treatment*

Compared with the extensive published data regarding the surgical management of TFCC injuries in adults, little has been written about the results of treatment in the pediatric patient population. Terry and Waters reviewed a series of 29 children and adolescents from the authors' institution treated for post-traumatic, surgically documented TFCC injuries [37]. All patients presented for evaluation of ulnar wrist pain, and approximately half had sustained a concomitant distal radius fracture at the initial injury. The average age was 13 years. More than three fourths of patients had Palmer 1B lesions. Eighty-six percent of patients had coexisting wrist pathology, most commonly ulnar styloid nonunion, DRUJ instability, distal radial fracture malunion, or ulnocarpal impaction in the setting of ulnar positive variance. All Palmer 1B, 1C, and 1D tears were repaired using the principles and techniques outlined here. At average follow-up of 21 months, more than 85% of patients had good to excellent results as assessed by the modified Mayo Wrist score [37,47,61].

## Summary

Management of distal radius fractures is guided by the pattern and location of injury, degree of deformity, and expectations of bony remodeling based on the amount of remaining skeletal growth. Indications for surgical treatment include unstable or irreducible fractures, open fractures, floating elbow injuries, and neurovascular or soft-tissue compromise precluding cast immobilization. Patients and families should be counseled regarding the potential for post-traumatic distal radial growth arrest following physeal fractures. In these cases, epiphysiodeses, ulnar shortening osteotomies, or corrective radial osteotomies may be performed, depending on the pattern of arrest, degree of deformity, and remaining skeletal growth.

TFCC tears may be the source of ulnar-sided wrist pain in children and adolescents, though symptoms and physical examination findings may be subtle. Patients who have persistent pain and functional limitations despite activity modification and therapy are candidates for surgical treatment. Appropriate repair of peripheral TFCC tears with correction of concomitant wrist pathology restores normal wrist anatomy, alleviates pain, and allows for return to functional activities.

## References

[1] Cheng JCY, Shen WY. Limb fracture pattern in different age groups: a study of 3,350 children J Orthop Trauma 1993;7:15–22.

[2] Landin LA. Fracture patterns in children. Acta Orthop Scand 1983;54(Suppl 202):1–109.

[3] Worlock P, Stower M. Fracture patterns in Nottingham children. J Pediatr Orthop [Am] 1986;6:656–60.

[4] Mann DC, Rajmaira S. Distribution of physeal and nonphyseal fractures of long bones in children aged 0 to 16 years. J Pediatr Orthop [Am] 1990;10:713–6.

[5] Chadwick CJ, Bentley G. The classification and prognosis of epiphyseal injuries. Injury 1987;18:157–68.

[6] Neer CS, Horwitz BS. Fractures of the proximal humeral epiphyseal plate. Clin Orthop 1965;41:24–31.

[7] Peterson HA, Madhok R, Benson JT, et al. Physeal fractures: part 1. Epidemiology in Olmsted County,

Minnesota, 1979–1988. J Pediatr Orthop [Am] 1994; 14:423–30.

[8] Boyd KT, Brownson P, Hunter JB. Distal radial fractures in young goalkeepers: a case for an appropriately sized soccer ball. [Br] J Sports Med 2001;35:409–11.

[9] Taylor BL, Attia MW. Sports-related injuries in children. Acad Emerg Med 2000;7:1376–82.

[10] Khosla S, Melton LJ, Dekutoski MB, et al. Incidence of childhood distal forearm fractures over 30 years: a population-based study. JAMA 2003;290:1479–85.

[11] Skaggs DL, Loro ML, Pitukcheewanont P, et al. Increased body weight and decreased radial cross-sectional dimensions in girls with forearm fractures. J Bone Miner Res 2001;16:1337–42.

[12] Friberg KS. Remodeling after distal forearm fractures in children. III. Correction of residual angulation in fractures of the radius. Acta Orthop Scand 1979;50:741–9.

[13] Houshian S, Holst AK, Larsen MS, et al. Remodeling of Salter-Harris type II epiphyseal plate injury of the distal radius. J Pediatr Orthop [Am] 2004;24:472–6.

[14] Younger ASE, Tredwell SJ, Mackenzie WG. Factors affecting fracture position at cast removal after pediatric forearm fracture. J Pediatr Orthop [Am] 1997;17:332–6.

[15] Zimmermann R, Gschwentner M, Pechlaner S, et al. Remodeling capacity and functional outcome of palmarly versus dorsally displaced pediatric radius fractures in the distal one-third. Arch Orthop Trauma Surg 2004;124:42–8.

[16] Johari AN, Sinha M. Remodeling of forearm fractures in children. J Pediatr Orthop [Br] 1999;8:84–7.

[17] Davidson JS, Brown DJ, Barnes SN, et al. Simple treatment for torus fractures of the distal radius. J Bone Joint Surg [Br] 2001;83:1173–5.

[18] Solan MC, Rees R, Daly K. Current management of torus fractures of the distal radius. Injury 2002;33:503–5.

[19] Symons S, Rowsell M, Bhowal B, et al. Hospital versus home management of children with buckle fractures of the distal radius. A prospective, randomized trial. J Bone Joint Surg [Br] 2001;83:556–60.

[20] West S, Andrews J, Bebbington A, et al. Buckle fractures of the distal radius are safely treated in a soft bandage: a randomized prospective trial of bandage versus plaster cast. J Pediatr Orthop [Am] 2005;25:322–5.

[21] Gibbons CL, Woods DA, Pailthorpe C, et al. The management of isolated distal radius fractures in children. J Pediatr Orthop [Am] 1994;14:207–10.

[22] Miller BS, Taylor B, Widmann RF, et al. Cast immobilization versus percutaneous pin fixation of displaced distal radius fractures in children: a prospective, randomized study. J Pediatr Orthop [Am] 2005;25:490–4.

[23] Proctor MT, Moore DJ, Paterson JM. Redisplacement after manipulation of distal radial fractures in children. J Bone Joint Surg [Br] 1993;75:453–4.

[24] Choi KY, Chan WS, Lam TP, et al. Percutaneous Kirschner-wire pinning for severely displaced distal radial fractures in children. A report of 157 cases. J Bone Joint Surg [Br] 1995;77:797–801.

[25] Ring D, Waters PM, Hotchkiss RN, et al. Pediatric floating elbow. J Pediatr Orthop [Am] 2001;21: 456–9.

[26] Waters PM, Kolettis GJ, Schwend R. Acute median neuropathy following physeal fractures of the distal radius. J Pediatr Orthop [Am] 1994;14:173–7.

[27] Yung PS, Lam CY, Ng BK, et al. Percutaneous transphyseal intramedullary Kirschner wire pinning: a safe and effective procedure for treatment of displaced diaphyseal forearm fracture in children. J Pediatr Orthop [Am] 2004;24:7–12.

[28] McLauchlan GJ, Cowan B, Annan IH, et al. Management of completely displaced metaphyseal fractures of the distal radius in children. A prospective, randomized controlled trial. J Bone Joint Surg [Br] 2002;84:413–7.

[29] Salter RB, Harris WR. Injuries involving the epiphyseal plate. J Bone Joint Surg [Am] 1963;45:587.

[30] Cannata G, DeMaio F, Mancini F, et al. Physeal fractures of the distal radius and ulna: long-term prognosis. J Orthop Trauma 2003;17:172–80.

[31] Horii E, Tamura Y, Nakamura R, et al. Premature closure of the distal radial physis. J Hand Surg [Br] 1993;18:11–6.

[32] Hove LM, Engesaeter LB. Corrective osteotomies after injuries of the distal radial physis in children. J Hand Surg [Br] 1997;22:699–704.

[33] Lee BS, Esterhai JL, Das M. Fracture of the distal radial epiphysis. Characteristic and surgical treatment of premature, post-traumatic epiphyseal closure. Clin Orthop 1984;185:90–6.

[34] Waters PM, Bae DS, Montgomery KD. Surgical management of posttraumatic distal radial growth arrest in adolescents. J Pediatr Orthop [Am] 2002; 22:717–24.

[35] Zehntner MK, Jakob RP, McGanity PL. Growth disturbance of the distal radial epiphysis after trauma: operative treatment by corrective radial osteotomy. J Pediatr Orthop [Am] 1990;10:411–5.

[36] Palmer AK, Werner FW. The triangular fibrocartilage complex of the wrist: anatomy and function. J Hand Surg [Am] 1981;6:153–62.

[37] Terry CL, Waters PM. Triangular fibrocartilage injuries in pediatric and adolescent patients. J Hand Surg [Am] 1998;23:626–34.

[38] Jones SJ, Lyons RA, Silbert J, et al. Changes in sports injuries to children between 1983 and 1998: comparison of case series. J Public Health Med 2001;23:268–71.

[39] Purvis JM, Burke RG. Recreational injuries in children: incidence and prevention. J Am Acad Orthop Surg 2001;9:365–74.

[40] Kato H, Nakamura R, Shionoya K, et al. Does high-resolution MR imaging have better accuracy than standard MR imaging for evaluation of the triangular fibrocartilage complex? J Hand Surg [Br] 2000; 25:487–91.

[41] Saupe N, Prussmann KP, Luechinger R, et al. MR imaging of the wrist: comparison between 1.5- and 3-T MR imaging—preliminary experience. Radiology 2005;234:256–64.

[42] Palmer AK, Werner FW. Biomechanics of the distal radioulnar joint. Clin Orthop 1984;187:26–35.

[43] Palmer AK. The distal radioulnar joint: anatomy, biomechanics, and triangular fibrocartilage complex abnormalities. Hand Clin 1987;3:31–40.

[44] Steyers CM, Blair WF. Measuring ulnar variance: a comparison of techniques. J Hand Surg [Am] 1989;14:607–12.

[45] Sugimoto H, Shinozaki T, Ohsawa T. Triangular fibrocartilage in asymptomatic subjects: investigation of abnormal MR signal intensity. Radiology 1994;191:193–7.

[46] Palmer AK. Triangular fibrocartilage complex lesions: a classification. J Hand Surg [Am] 1989;14: 594–606.

[47] Cooney WP, Linscheid RL, Dobyns JH. Triangular fibrocartilage tears. J Hand Surg [Am] 1994;19: 143–54.

[48] Buterbaugh GA. Radiocarpal arthroscopy portals and normal anatomy. Hand Clin 1994;10:567–76.

[49] de Araujo W, Poehling GG, Kuzma GR. New Tuohy needle technique for triangular fibrocartilage complex repair: preliminary studies. Arthroscopy 1996; 12:699–703.

[50] Whipple TL, Geissler WB. Arthroscopic management of wrist triangular fibrocartilage complex injuries in the athlete. Orthopedics 1993;16: 1061–7.

[51] McAdams TR, Hentz VR. Injury to the dorsal sensory branch of the ulnar nerve in the arthroscopic repair of ulnar-sided triangular fibrocartilage tears using an inside-out technique: a cadaver study. J Hand Surg [Am] 2002;27:840–4.

[52] Trumble TE, Gilbert M, Vedder N. Isolated tears of the triangular fibrocartilage: management by early arthroscopic repair. J Hand Surg [Am] 1997;22: 57–65.

[53] Zachee B, DeSmet L, Fabry G. Arthroscopic suturing of TFCC lesions. Arthroscopy 1993;9:242–3.

[54] Adams BD. Distal radioulnar joint instability. In: Green DP, Hotchkiss RN, Pederson WC, et al, editors. Green's operative hand surgery. 5th edition. Philadelphia: Elsevier; 2005. p. 605–44.

[55] Skie MC, Mekhail AO, Deitrich DR, et al. Operative technique for inside-out repair of the triangular fibrocartilage complex. J Hand Surg [Am] 1997;22: 814–7.

[56] Trumble TE, Culp R, Hanel DP, et al. Intra-articular fractures of the distal aspect of the radius. J Bone Joint Surg [Am] 1998;80:582–600.

[57] Hauck RM, Skahen J, Palmer AK. Classification and treatment of ulnar styloid nonunion. J Hand Surg [Am] 1996;21:418–22.

[58] Feldon P, Terrono AL, Belsky MR. Wafer distal ulna resection for triangular fibrocartilage tears and/or ulna impaction syndrome. J Hand Surg [Am] 1992;17:731–7.

[59] Minami A, Kato H. Ulnar shortening osteotomy for triangular fibrocartilage complex tears associated with ulnar positive variance. J Hand Surg [Am] 1998;23:904–8.

[60] Trumble TE, Gilbert M, Vedder N. Ulnar shortening combined with arthroscopic repairs in the delayed management of triangular fibrocartilage complex tears. J Hand Surg [Am] 1997;22:807–13.

[61] Cooney WP, Bussey R, Dobyns JH, et al. Difficult wrist fractures: perilunate fracture-dislocations of the wrist. Clin Orthop 1987;214:136–47.

ELSEVIER
SAUNDERS

Hand Clin 22 (2006) 55–67

HAND
CLINICS

# Forearm Fractures in Children and Adolescents: A Practical Approach

Martin J. Herman, MD*, Silas T. Marshall, BA

*Department of Orthopedic Surgery, Division of Pediatric Orthopedics, Drexel University College of Medicine,
St. Christopher's Hospital for Children, 3601 A Street, Philadelphia, PA 19134, USA*

Children and adolescents who sustain displaced fractures of the radius and ulna are best treated primarily with closed reduction of the fracture and cast immobilization. Outcomes for treatment with nonsurgical methods are excellent in most cases. Because of a lack of evidence-based research, operative indications are controversial. Opinions vary regarding acceptable radiographic parameters of reduction. Clinical outcomes do not correlate strictly with fracture alignment at healing [1,2]. In the past decade, a trend toward more frequent use of surgery for management of displaced forearm fractures has emerged [3]. This article presents a practical approach to management of displaced radius and ulna fractures in children and adolescents while addressing areas of controversy. Nonsurgical and surgical management are discussed. A technique for intramedullary fixation of the radius and ulna is presented in detail.

## Epidemiology

Diaphyseal fractures of the radius and ulna account for approximately 5% of all children's fractures [4]. These injuries occur more commonly in boys than in girls and the nondominant arm is fractured more frequently. Boys sustain these injuries at two different median age peaks, age 9 years and age 14 years, and girls sustain these injuries at a median age of 9 years [5]. Most forearm fractures occur as isolated injuries of the

extremity; associated disruption of the radiocapitellar joint (Monteggia fracture and equivalents) and the distal radioulnar joint (Galeazzi fracture and equivalents) and other complex injury patterns occur infrequently.

## Mechanism of injury

Forearm fractures are caused most commonly by indirect forces, predominantly falls onto an outstretched arm; falls from playground equipment, bicycles, or trees are also common etiologies. On impact, the loading force is first transmitted through the radius, which fails first, followed by the ulna [6]. Associated torsional forces dictate the specific fracture type, pattern, and displacement. Higher energy trauma, such as auto–pedestrian injuries and child abuse [7], are less common. Direct forces may cause isolated fractures of the radius or ulna and both-bone injuries.

## Fracture level and pattern

Approximately 75% of fractures of the radius and ulna occur in the distal one third of the forearm, 15% in the middle one third, and 5% in the proximal one third [8]. Younger children sustain fractures more commonly in the middle one third of the forearm. Older children's injuries tend to occur more distally. The radius fracture is proximal to the ulna fracture in most children and adolescents. Complete transverse or short oblique fractures with little or no comminution are the most common fracture types; plastic deformation (Fig. 1) and greenstick injuries are seen more commonly in younger children.

\* Corresponding author.
*E-mail address:* Martin1.herman@tenethealth.com
(M.J. Herman).

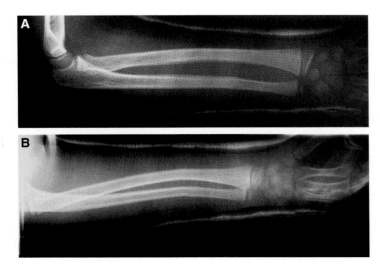

Fig. 1. (A) Anterior-posterior (AP) and lateral (B) radiographs of a 5-year-old boy who fell from the monkey bars. Although the AP view seems normal, he has a plastic deformity of the radius and ulna with 15° of apex volar angulation. He was treated with 6 weeks of cast immobilization; no reduction was required.

### Pertinent anatomy

The radius is cylindric in its proximal third and triangular-shaped in the middle third. As the radius transitions from diaphyseal to metaphyseal bone distally, it becomes more rectangular-shaped and flattened on its volar and dorsal surfaces. The radius has a lateral bow that begins just distal to the bicipital tuberosity with an apex at approximately midshaft. Physes are located proximally and distally; 75% of longitudinal growth occurs distally. The bicipital tuberosity is anteromedial on the radius just distal to the proximal physis. Lister's tubercle is dorsal on the metaphysis just proximal to the distal physis. These landmarks are not radiographically evident in younger children.

The proximal ulna is triangular-shaped but becomes more cylindric in the mid-diaphysis and distally. The ulna is essentially straight with the exception of a 10° to 15° apex radial bow in the proximal end. The olecranon apophysis at the proximal end begins to ossify at approximately age 10 years. The distal ulnar physis contributes more than 80% to longitudinal growth. The radius and ulna are attached proximally by the annular ligament, throughout the diaphysis by the interosseous membrane, and distally by the ligaments of the distal radioulnar joint and triangular fibrocartilage complex. Forearm rotation occurs as the radius rotates around the ulna, facilitated by the radial bow and the mobility of the interosseous membrane, which contains multiple components that vary in tightness with forearm rotation.

### Clinical evaluation

The diagnosis of a forearm fracture in a child or adolescent is generally obvious. The child or adolescent presents with swelling, pain, and deformity in the injured extremity after trauma. Point tenderness and bony crepitus are common clinical findings in children who have displaced, complete fractures. Those children who have minimally displaced complete fractures, greenstick fractures, and plastic deformation are identified less easily. Because of thick periosteum, fracture fragment mobility is limited. Younger, nonverbal children may only display discomfort with upper extremity weightbearing during crawling or other activities; minor swelling and limited active and passive movement of the arm may be the only clinical signs.

On clinical examination, limb deformity and the degree of swelling within the compartments noted. The skin is inspected for lacerations, abrasions, and signs of intentional injury. Perfusion of the arm is assessed by palpation of the pulses and evaluation of capillary refill. Motor and sensory testing of median, ulnar, and radial nerves must be performed and properly documented. This examination is notoriously difficult in young children. To complete the evaluation, a thorough examination of the entire injured extremity, from the shoulder to the hand, is mandatory to diagnose associated proximal or distal joint disruptions of the forearm and other ipsilateral injuries.

## Primary treatment

In the emergency department, the child's forearm is splinted provisionally after gentle re-alignment to allow for adequate, comfortable radiographic evaluation. High quality anterior-posterior (AP) and lateral radiographs of the forearm, elbow, and wrist are necessary to assess fully the extent of the injury. Before attempting closed reduction, the surgeon must identify the level of the fracture of each bone, the degree of completeness of each fracture, the direction and degree of angulation and malrotation, the degree of shortening, and associated injuries of the elbow and wrist joints.

## Technique of closed reduction

Closed reduction generally is performed in the emergency department under conscious sedation. For incomplete fractures, correction of rotational deformity and manual reduction of angulation without traction is used to realign these injuries in most cases [9]. Some investigators advocate completions of the greenstick fracture to prevent re-angulation [10] or to diminish the risk for re-fracture [11]. Others [9,12], including the authors, believe that the intact cortex aids in achieving and maintaining alignment, and therefore do not purposely complete the greenstick fracture. Fractures with apex volar angulation are reduced by supinating the forearm and applying a dorsally-directed force at the apex. Fractures presenting with apex dorsal angulation are reduced in the opposite fashion. After reduction, a long arm splint or cast is applied with the elbow flexed to 90° and the forearm positioned in neutral rotation.

Complete fractures present a more considerable challenge. The diaphyseal fracture fragments are subject to the muscle forces of the forearm that produce predictable patterns of displacement, malrotation, and shortening based on fracture location (Fig. 2). Understanding these deforming forces aids the surgeon in achieving satisfactory reduction. First, longitudinal traction is applied by grasping the forearm distal to the fracture or hand while countertraction is applied proximally to the forearm or to the distal humerus by an

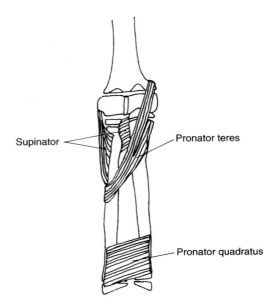

Supinator — Pronator teres

Pronator quadratus

Fig. 2. The muscle forces on the fracture fragments determine the rotational position of the proximal fragment. Knowledge of these forces assists the surgeon in achieving an acceptable rotational reduction. With a fracture of the proximal third of the radius the supinator muscle pulls the proximal fragment into supination. With a fracture of the distal third of the radius the pronator quadratus pulls the distal fragment into pronation. Midshaft fractures generally lie in neutral rotation. (Courtesy of Silas T. Marshall, BA, Philadelphia, PA.)

assistant. Alternatively, the extremity may be placed in finger traps (Fig. 3); distraction force is applied manually or by suspension of a light weight on the distal humerus. Next, the fracture fragments are manipulated to reduce angulation and, if possible, to achieve end-to-end bony contact without overriding. Traction may promote spontaneous rotational reduction [13]. In general, fractures of the proximal one third of the forearm are best realigned by supinating the forearm. Fractures of the middle one third are reduced with the forearm in neutral rotation. Fractures of the distal one third are reduced best in pronation. Extreme rotational positioning greater than 30° to 40°, especially extreme pronation, is not recommended, to reduce the risk for loss of forearm rotation after fracture healing from contracture of the interosseous membrane.

A long arm cast or splint is applied after reduction. Bulky padding must be avoided. Three-point molding around the fracture site and anterior–posterior molding of the forearm in its middle one third to achieve separation of the radius

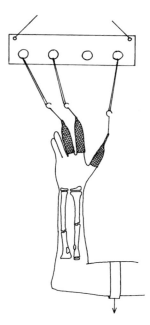

Fig. 3. Finger traps are useful to provide longitudinal traction while attempting closed reduction. After application of a small weight or manual traction on the humerus, the fracture fragments are manipulated. The cast or splint is applied with the hand suspended in the finger traps. (Courtesy of Christopher A. Samujh, BA, Philadelphia, PA.)

and ulna and to maintain the interosseous space are crucial for maintenance of reduction. The ideal cast or sugar-tong splint, when dry, is oval-shaped when viewed laterally at the mid-forearm, with slight depressions of the plaster or fiberglass where three-point molding was applied. When applying a cast, flattening of the ulnar and posterior humeral borders and supracondylar molding assist in preventing migration of the extremity in the cast, a common mechanism of reduction loss, especially in younger children. Although immobilization of the elbow at 90° of flexion is recommended for most fractures, maintenance of the elbow in extension and incorporation of the thumb in the cast to prevent distal cast migration may be useful for some proximal forearm fractures [14].

*Acceptable reduction*

After reduction and splinting or casting, repeat AP and lateral radiographs of the forearm are evaluated. Alignment of the radius and ulna are measured on the AP and lateral radiographs to define angulation. Malrotation is difficult to assess. A mismatch of cortical diameter as measured on

either side of the fracture site is a qualitative method of assessment for malrotation. Identifying the position of the radial tuberosity on the AP radiograph allows for a quantitative measure of the degree of proximal fragment rotation; the degree of malrotation then can be determined by comparing the clinical position of the distal forearm with this measurement [15]. The degree of shortening is best measured on the lateral radiograph.

The parameters that constitute an acceptable reduction of the radius and ulna are controversial. Guidelines based on published reports vary regarding the acceptable degree of angulation, malrotation, and shortening that will yield satisfactory clinical outcomes for a child of a given age. As opposed to the adult, the growing child who has at least 2 years of growth remaining has the capacity for remodeling of residual deformity. Remodeling may be dramatic (Fig. 4). Remodeling occurs most reliably in younger children who have more distal fractures and deformity in the sagittal plane [16,17]. Proximal one-third angulation, rotational malunion, and flattening of the radial bow remodel less predictably, particularly in children older than 10 years of age [2,18].

Adding to the controversy is evidence that radiographic malunion does not correlate absolutely with future forearm rotation and clinical function [8,13]. Some children who have residual forearm angulation as much as 15° and partial loss of forearm rotation are unaware of their functional deficits [2,17]. Furthermore, achievement of acceptable position at fracture healing by closed methods [19] or by surgery does not guarantee full return of forearm rotation [20].

In the authors' opinion, the guidelines of Noonan and Price [21] are best for making clinical judgments. For children younger than 9 years of age, 15° of angulation, 45° of malrotation, and complete overriding of the fragments are acceptable parameters of reduction. For children older than 9 years of age with fractures of the middle and distal one thirds of the forearm, 15° of angulation, 30° of malrotation, and complete overriding are acceptable radiographic parameters; no more than 10° of angulation with similar degrees of malrotation and overriding is acceptable for children older than 9 years of age who have fractures of the proximal one third.

*Care after reduction*

If the reduction is within acceptable limits, the child is discharged from the emergency department

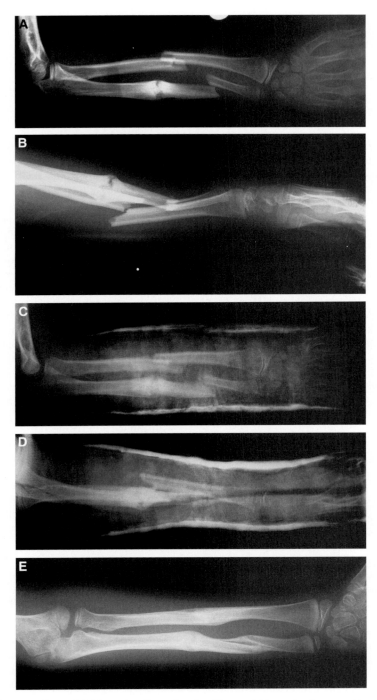

Fig. 4. (A) Anterior-posterior and (B) lateral radiographs of a 10-year-old boy who 1 year earlier underwent open reduction and internal fixation of the radius and ulna with intramedullary smooth wires. He sustained a refracture at the
radial site and a new fracture distal to the old ulnar fracture site. His previous ulnar fracture site had incomplete radiographic healing but was asymptomatic. After closed reduction in the emergency department, he was placed in a long arm
cast (C and D) for a total of 10 weeks. At 4-month follow-up from injury he had 50° pronation and 60° supination with
no deformity. His radiographs (E and F) show extensive remodeling.

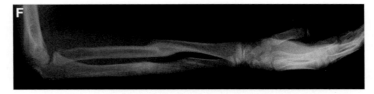

Fig. 4 (*continued*)

after awakening from sedation and a re-evaluation of the neurovascular status. Children who have severe swelling or an abnormal examination after reduction and immobilization should be admitted for observation. Weekly clinical and radiographic follow-up is recommended for the first 3 weeks after injury to confirm maintenance of reduction. Repeat closed manipulation of forearm fractures that show loss of alignment in follow-up may be done successfully under anesthesia within 2 to 3 weeks after injury in younger children and occasionally up to 4 weeks in older children. Cast immobilization is discontinued after 6 to 8 weeks when clinical examination and radiographs indicate healing. Older children may require 8 to 10 weeks of immobilization. Children are permitted to resume activities within 4 to 6 weeks after cast removal in most cases. Physical therapy may be necessary for some older children but is not prescribed routinely.

### Surgical management

#### Indications

Most children who have fractures of the forearm may be treated successfully with closed reduction and cast immobilization. Primary surgical reduction with fracture fixation is best indicated for open fractures [22,23], fractures that occur in association with severe soft tissue injury or compartment syndrome, and fractures that occur in association with ipsilateral fractures of the distal humerus (floating elbow) [24]. Surgical reduction and fixation also is indicated for fractures that cannot be manipulated initially into acceptable alignment by closed means (aka, irreducible fracture) and for those fractures that have lost alignment in the cast at follow-up and have failed repeat closed reduction.

#### Intramedullary fixation

The following important differences exist between the growing child and the adult who has a displaced fracture of the forearm: (1) children have the capacity for some remodeling. Achieving anatomic alignment after fracture is not crucial to a successful outcome; maintenance of acceptable reduction parameters alone is the goal of fixation; (2) in general, children's diaphyseal fractures heal more reliably and quickly compared with adults; delayed union and nonunion of closed fractures are rare; fracture site compression is not necessary to achieve union after closed or open reduction; (3) thick periosteum and incomplete fracture patterns prevent severe fracture displacement; and (4) closed manipulation or open reduction through a limited surgical approach is successful in restoring fracture alignment in most cases.

For these reasons, intramedullary fixation is the best treatment choice for growing children who have forearm fractures that require surgery [25–27]. Smooth wires or flexible titanium nails may be introduced into the intramedullary canal with limited dissection and advanced across the fracture site after a closed or a limited open fracture reduction. These implants reliably maintain alignment, serving as internal splints during healing in a cast. An additional advantage is that these devices may be removed in the office or during a short surgical procedure with less morbidity and risk for refracture compared with plate removal [28,29].

#### Technique of intramedullary fixation

After induction of general anesthesia, the child is positioned with the effected extremity lying on a radiolucent hand table. Confirmation that the entire forearm may be visualized by fluoroscopy before draping is recommended. After placement of a tourniquet on the upper arm, the entire extremity distal to the tourniquet is prepped and draped in a sterile fashion to allow access to the elbow, forearm, and hand. Ulnar fracture reduction and fixation generally is accomplished more easily and is performed first. To minimize the tourniquet time, ulna reduction and fixation may be done safely with the tourniquet deflated.

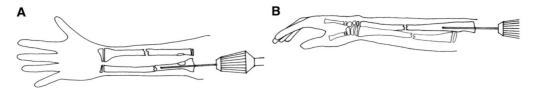

Fig. 5. (*A*) and (*B*) Fixation of the ulna is accomplished by anterograde drilling of a smooth wire through the tip of the olecranon. Alternatively, a precontoured smooth wire or flexible titanium nail may be introduced into the intramedullary canal after pre-drilling a small entry hole and manually advancing the implant with a T-handled chuck. (Courtesy of Christopher A. Samujh, BA, Philadelphia, PA.)

A small incision is made first over the tip of the olecranon process. Under fluoroscopic guidance, a smooth wire (0.062 or 5/64th size) is drilled across the olecranon apophysis and into the intramedullary canal. Alternatively, a flexible titanium nail (2.0–2.5 mm diameter) or a smooth wire (0.062 or 5/64th size) precontoured with a 30° bend approximately 5 mm proximal to its blunt end, is introduced into the intramedullary canal through a hole drilled under fluoroscopy in the proximal ulna (Fig. 5). The extramedullary part of the implant then is inserted into a drill or, for precontoured implants, a T-handled chuck, and advanced anterograde to the fracture site. Using traction and closed manipulation at the fracture site, the ulna fracture is realigned under fluoroscopy. Avoidance of excessive and forceful closed manipulation lessens the iatrogenic damage to already swollen and traumatized soft tissues.

Conversion of the closed reduction to an open treatment is recommended after no more than 10 minutes of manipulation. When open reduction is necessary, the fracture site is best approached along the subcutaneous ulnar border through a 2- to 3-cm incision. After fracture site exposure, two bone-holding forceps are applied at opposite sides of the fracture. The fracture is reduced manually by the surgeon under direct vision while an assistant provides longitudinal traction and rotational control of the distal fragment.

After successful reduction, the smooth wire is drilled across the fracture site or, for precontoured implants, advanced by gentle manual forward pressure while rotating the T-handled chuck through a small arc of motion to prevent binding on the cortex and inadvertent perforation. The distal tip of the implant then is advanced to the metaphysis of the distal ulna. For fractures of the distal one third of the ulna, additional fixation of the distal ulnar fragment may be achieved by drilling the smooth wire into the metaphysis, physis, or distal epiphysis; a precontoured implant cannot be advanced beyond the metaphysis. The proximal end of the implant is bent at the olecranon tip and left percutaneous or is cut and buried beneath the skin. The later method is preferred, especially when ulnar open reduction is necessary.

After reduction and fixation of the ulna, the radius fracture is addressed. The limb is exsanguinated and the tourniquet is inflated. A 1-cm longitudinal incision is made over the dorsal radius

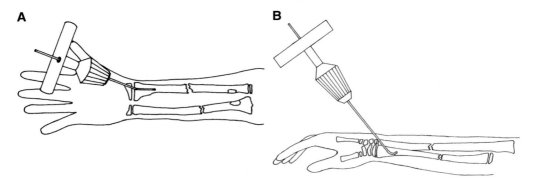

Fig. 6. (*A*) The radial implant is inserted through a small drill hole made approximately 1 cm proximal to the distal radial physis. (*B*) Care must be taken to avoid penetration of the volar radial cortex when advancing the implant proximally. (Courtesy of Christopher A. Samujh, BA, Philadelphia, PA.)

1 cm proximal to the distal radial physis in the midline of the metaphysis at approximately Lister tubercle. In younger children the tubercle is not palpable and fluoroscopy may be necessary to identify the incision site. After skin incision, the dorsal retinaculum is incised and the interval between the third and fourth dorsal compartments is divided, exposing the metaphysis of the distal radius. After verifying position with fluoroscopy, a unicortical drill hole is made while protecting the soft tissues with a drill sleeve; the hole is enlarged by gradually directing the drill in a proximal direction at a 30° angle from the dorsal shaft. A precontoured smooth wire or flexible titanium nail may be used for radial fixation. For fractures at the apex of the radial bow, a flexible titanium nail contoured to match the radial bow of the child's forearm is recommended. After insertion into the T-handled chuck, the implant is introduced into the dorsal drill hole under direct vision to avoid tendon laceration or entrapment (Fig. 6). By applying manual forward pressure to the T-handled chuck, the implant is advanced retrograde to the fracture site; care must be taken to avoid

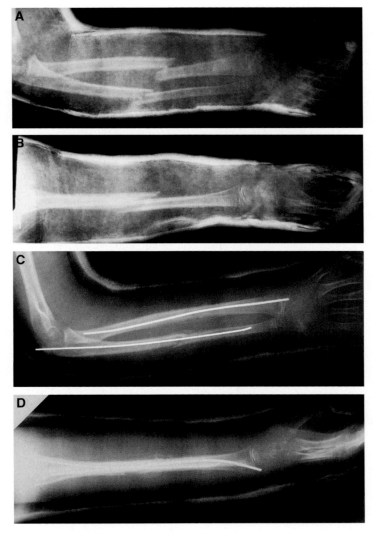

Fig. 7. (*A*) Anterior-posterior and (*B*) lateral radiographs of a 10.5-year-old girl who underwent two previous closed reductions under anesthesia; she is 2 weeks after a fall from her bicycle. She underwent open reduction and internal fixation of the radius and ulna with intramedullary smooth wire fixation (*C* and *D*).

perforation of the volar cortex. After passage of the implant to the radial fracture site, closed reduction is attempted. As with reduction of the ulna, conversion to an open procedure is recommended after no more than 10 minutes of closed manipulation.

Open reduction of middle and distal radial shaft fractures generally is best done through a dorsal approach; fractures of the proximal one third are best exposed by way of a volar approach. Exposure that allows for safe application of bone-holding forceps proximal and distal to the fracture site and direct visualization of the reduction is all that is necessary. Generally the incision and exposure are less extensive than that required for plate application. After open fracture realignment, the implant is advanced retrograde across the fracture site to the metaphysis of the proximal radius. For fractures at apex of the radial bow, the rod is rotated after insertion under fluoroscopic visualization until the position that best restores the radial bow is identified. The extramedullary end of the implant then is bent and cut outside the skin or is cut and buried beneath the skin. The latter technique is the preferred method to avoid dorsal skin irritation under the cast (see Fig. 7).

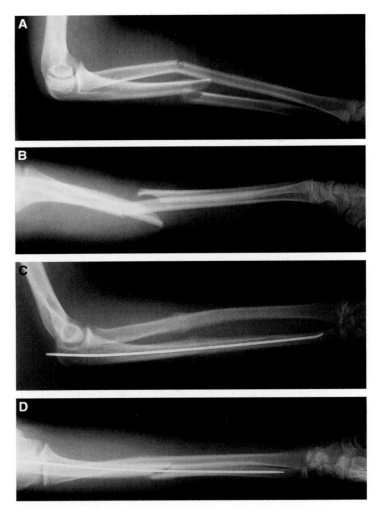

Fig. 8. (*A*) Anterior-posterior and (*B*) lateral radiographs of a 14-year-old boy who fell onto an outstretched hand while wrestling. He sustained a grade 1 open fracture of the ulna and a greenstick fracture of the radius. After irrigation and debridement of the open wound, he underwent open reduction and internal fixation of the ulna. A 2.5-mm titanium elastic nail was used to stabilize the ulna. The radius fracture was reduced closed (*C* and *D*).

## Care after surgery

After completion of surgery, a bivalved long arm cast or sugar-tong splint is applied; after 1 week the bivalved cast is made circumferential or the splint is converted to a cast. Cast immobilization is continued for 8 to 12 weeks. Implants left outside the skin are removed in the office after no longer than 6 weeks. Buried implants are removed in the operating room 8 to 16 weeks after surgery. Children are permitted to resume activities within 4 to 6 weeks after cast removal in most cases. Physical therapy may be necessary for some older children but is not prescribed commonly.

## Other surgical considerations

### Single bone fixation

Fixation of the ulna (see Fig. 8) or radius (see Fig. 9) is an option for some both-bone forearm fractures in children and adolescents [30–32]. An intramedullary implant or plate is applied to one bone and closed reduction of the other bone is performed. In the authors' experience, this technique is most successful for managing forearm fractures in which one bone has an incomplete fracture (greenstick or plastic deformation) or a complete fracture that is reduced readily while the other bone cannot be maintained in alignment by cast immobilization or is irreducible. Postoperative immobilization in a carefully molded long arm cast is mandatory to maintain acceptable reduction when single bone fixation is used to treat displaced fractures of the radius and ulna. Inadequate immobilization may result in loss of reduction of the bone without fixation.

### Plate fixation

Plate fixation for children's forearm fractures is indicated only for those fractures with comminution or those located at the apex of the radial bow that cannot be maintained in alignment by intramedullary fixation. Older children and adolescents with closed distal radial and ulnar physes regardless of chronologic age are treated as adults with plate fixation. A third tubular plate or 2.4-mm compression plate (3–5-hole length) is adequate to maintain reduction and achieve union in most children. Larger 3.5-mm compression plates are reserved for the older child and adolescent who has bone of sufficient size to allow placement of these implants.

### External fixation

External fixation using 3.5-mm or smaller screws placed under direct vision is used only for

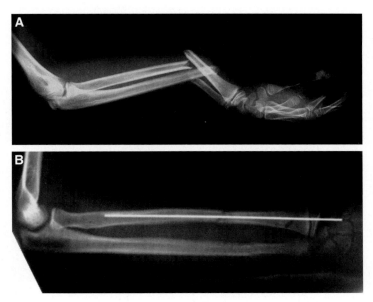

Fig. 9. (*A*) Radiograph of a 7-year-old girl who was struck by a motor vehicle while on her bicycle. She sustained a grade 2 open fracture of the radius. After irrigation and debridement she underwent open reduction and intramedullary fixation of the radius only (*B*).

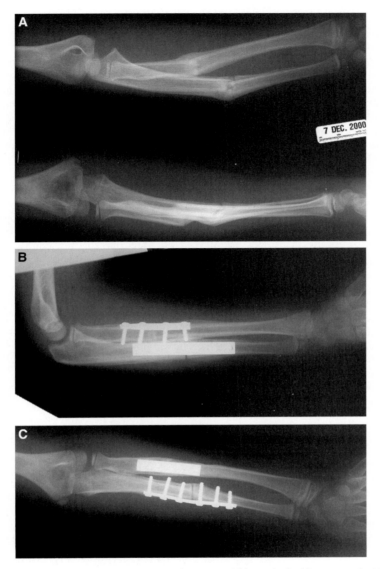

Fig. 10. (*A*) Anterior-posterior and lateral radiographs of a 9-year-old boy who had been treated with 10 weeks of cast immobilization. He had a deformity of the forearm with minimal rotation 8 weeks after cast removal. He underwent osteotomies of the radius and ulna. Fixation was achieved with third tubular stainless steel plates (*B* and *C*).

those injuries associated with severe contamination, soft tissue loss or damage, and segmental bone loss that preclude use of other implants. External fixation may be used for short-term stabilization (less than 2 weeks) until the condition of the soft tissues is improved enough to permit conversion to other implants, or it may be used for definitive fracture management. This technique is rarely necessary for management of children's forearm fractures.

## Complications

### Malunion

Remodeling of fractures that heal with excessive angulation is unpredictable, and radiographic alignment does not absolutely predict forearm rotation or limb function. Children who have acceptable appearance and at least 30° of pronation and supination regardless of the degree of angulation generally have satisfactory clinical outcomes. Those who have unacceptable deformity and severely restricted motion after malunion are best treated with corrective osteotomy done within 1 year of fracture healing. For single plane deformities, drill osteoclasis [33] or osteotomy performed through a limited exposure and intramedullary fixation are adequate to restore and maintain realignment. Carefully planned corrective osteotomies held with plate fixation are recommended for complex malunions [34] (see Fig. 10). Although most children show improved rotation after realignment, a loss of rotation may occur after surgery.

*Refracture*

Refracture through a radiographically and clinically healed forearm fracture occurs in approximately 5% of children [2], generally within 6 months of the original injury. Management of these injuries follows guidelines for the primary injury (see Fig. 4). Achieving and maintaining alignment by closed reduction and cast immobilization is more difficult after refracture and outcomes are less predictable [2]. For those fractures that require fixation, closed passage of intramedullary fixation may not be possible if the intramedullary canal has not remodeled since the primary fracture; plate fixation is often necessary.

*Synostosis*

Synostosis of the radius and ulna is rare and occurs most frequently after proximal one third forearm fractures [35]. Fractures in children who have an associated head injury and fractures that result from high-energy trauma are at highest risk for developing a synostosis [36]. Multiple manipulations of the fracture to achieve reduction, surgical approaches to the radius and ulna made through a single incision, and wire fixation that spans the radius and ulna should be avoided to lessen the risk for synostosis. Restoration of forearm rotation by surgical takedown of the synostosis is unpredictable and re-synostosis does occur frequently [36].

*Complications of intramedullary fixation*

The risk for complications is increased for those children who undergo operative treatment of forearm fractures compared with those treated by closed reduction and cast immobilization [37]. Hardware migration and skin irritation, infection, and nerve injuries are the most common surgical complications [23,38,39]. Loss of reduction after

implant removal or that caused by implant deformation and delayed union also occur. Compartment syndrome after surgery also has been reported [40], and its occurrence most closely correlates with increased fluoroscopic use during surgery. Careful attention to implant insertion, maintenance of implants beneath the skin for a minimum of 8 to 12 weeks, and careful handling of soft tissue, especially while attempting reduction, may diminish the development of some of these complications.

## Acknowledgments

The authors thank Christopher A. Samujh, student of medicine, of Drexel University College of Medicine for his contribution of original artwork to this publication.

## References

[1] Hogstrom H, Nilsson BE, Willner S. Correction with growth following diaphyseal forearm fracture. Acta Orthop Scand 1976;47(3):299–303.
[2] Price CT, Scott DS, Kurzner ME, et al. Malunited forearm fractures in children. J Pediatr Orthop 1990; 10(6):705–12.
[3] Cheng JC, Ng BK, Ying SY, et al. A 10 year study of the changes in the pattern and treatment of 6,493 fractures. J Pediatr Orthop 1999;19(3):344–50.
[4] Landin LA. Fracture patterns in children. Acta Pediatr Scand Suppl 1983;54:192.
[5] Landin LA. Fracture patterns in children: Analysis of 8628 fractures with special reference to incidence, etiology, and secular changes in a Swedish urban population, 1950–1979. Acta Orthop Scand Suppl 1983;202:1–109.
[6] Treadwell SJ, Peteghem KV, Clough M. Pattern of forearm fractures in children. J Pediatr Orthop 1984;4(5):604–8.
[7] King J, Diefendorf D, Apthorp J, et al. Analysis of 429 fractures in 189 battered children. J Pediatr Orthop 1988;8(5):585–9.
[8] Thomas EM, Tuson KW, Browne PS. Fractures of the radius and ulna in children. Injury 1975;7(2): 120–4.
[9] Davis DR, Green DP. Forearm fractures in children: pitfalls and complications. Clin Orthop Rel Res 1976;120:172–83.
[10] Rang M. Children's fractures. Philadelphia: JB Lippincott; 1983.
[11] Gruber R. The problem of the relapse fracture in children. In: Chapchal G, editor. Fractures in children. Stuttgart: Georg Thieme Verlag; 1981. p. 154–8.
[12] Alpar EK, Thompson K, Owen R. Midshaft fractures of forearm bones in children. Injury 1981;13: 153–8.

[13] Carey PJ, Alburger PD, Betz RR, et al. Both-bone forearm fractures in children. Orthopedics 1992; 15(9):1015–9.

[14] Walker JL, Rang M. Forearm fractures in children: cast treatment with the elbow extended. J Bone Joint Surg [Br] 1991;73(2):299–301.

[15] Evans EM. Fractures of the radius and ulna. J Bone Joint Surg [Br] 1951;33:548–61.

[16] Younger ASE, Treadwell SJ, Mackenzie WG, et al. Accurate prediction of outcome after pediatric forearm fracture. J Pediatr Orthop 1994;14(2):200–6.

[17] Daruwalla JS. A study of radioulnar movements following fractures of the forearm in children. Clin Orthop 1979;139:114–20.

[18] Zionts LE, Zalavras C, Gerhardt MB. Closed treatment of displaced diaphyseal both-bone forearm fractures in older children and adolescents. J Pediatr Orthop 2005;25(4):507–12.

[19] Nilsson BE, Obrant K. The range of motion following fracture of the shaft of the forearm in children. Acta Orthop Scand 1977;48:600–2.

[20] Cullen MC, Roy DR, Giza E, et al. Complications of intramedullary fixation of pediatric forearm fractures. J Pediatr Orthop 1998;18(1):14–21.

[21] Noonen KJ, Price CT. Forearm and distal radius fractures in children. J Am Acad Orthop Surg 1998;6(3):146–56.

[22] Greenbaum B, Zionts LE, Ebramzadeh E. Open fractures of the forearm in children. J Orthop Trauma 2001;15(2):111–8.

[23] Luhmann SJ, Schootman M, Schoenecker PL, et al. Complications and outcomes of open pediatric forearm fractures. J Pediatr Orthop 2004;24(1):1–6.

[24] Ring D, Waters PM, Hotchkiss RN, et al. Pediatric floating elbow. J Pediatr Orthop 2001;21(4):456–9.

[25] Lascombes P, Prevot J, Ligier JN, et al. Elastic stable intramedullary nailing in forearm shaft fractures in children: 85 cases. J Pediatr Orthop 1990;10(2):167–71.

[26] Lee S, Nicol RO, Stott NS. Intramedullary fixation for pediatric unstable forearm fractures. Clin Orthop 2002;402:245–50.

[27] Richter D, Ostermann PAW, Ekkernkamp A, et al. Elastic intramedullary nailing: a minimally invasive concept in the treatment of unstable forearm fractures in children. J Pediatr Orthop 1998;18(4):457–61.

[28] Beaupre GS, Csongradi JJ. Refracture risk after plate removal in the forearm. J Orthop Trauma 1996;10(2):87–92.

[29] Nielson AB, Simonsen O. Displaced forearm fractures in children treated with AO plates. Injury 1984;15(6):393–6.

[30] Kirkos JM, Beslikas T, Kapras EA, et al. Surgical treatment of unstable diaphyseal both-bone forearm fractures in children with single fixation of the radius. Injury 2000;31(8):591–6.

[31] Flynn JM, Waters PM. Single-bone fixation of both-bone forearm fractures. J Pediatr Orthop 1996;16(5):655–9.

[32] Bhaskar AR, Roberts JA. Treatment of unstable fractures of the forearm in children: is plating of a single bone adequate? J Bone Joint Surg [Br] 2001;83B(2):253–8.

[33] Blount WP. Osteoclasis of the upper extremity in children. Acta Orthop Scand 1962;32:374–82.

[34] Trousdale RT, Linscheid RL. Operative treatment of malunited fractures of the forearm. J Bone Joint Surg [Am] 1995;77(6):894–902.

[35] Vince KG, Miller JE. Cross-union complicating fractures of the forearm. Part I: adults. J Bone Joint Surg [Am] 1987;69(5):640–53.

[36] Vince KG, Miller JE. Cross-union complicating fracture of the forearm. Part II: children. J Bone Joint Surg [Am] 1987;69(5):654–61.

[37] Smith VA, Goodman HJ, Strongwater A, et al. Treatment of pediatric both-bone forearm fractures: a comparison of operative techniques. J Pediatr Orthop 2005;25(3):309–13.

[38] Shoemaker SD, Comstock CP, Mubarak SJ, et al. Intramedullary Kirschner wire fixation of open or unstable forearm fractures in children. J Pediatr Orthop 1999;19(3):329–37.

[39] Luhmann SJ, Gordon JE, Schoenecker PL. Intramedullary fixation of unstable both-bone forearm fractures in children. J Pediatr Orthop 1998;18(4):451–6.

[40] Yuan PS, Pring ME, Gaynor TP, et al. Compartment syndrome following intramedullary fixation of pediatric forearm fractures. J Pediatr Orthop 2004;24(4):370–5.

ELSEVIER
SAUNDERS

Hand Clin 22 (2006) 69–75

# Pediatric Supracondylar Humerus Fractures

Mark Baratz, MD*, Chad Micucci, MD, Mark Sangimino, MD

*Allegheny Orthopedic Associates, 1307 Federal Street, 2nd Floor, Pittsburgh, PA 15212, USA*

A newly minted orthopedist gets a call from a physician in the local emergency department: "We have a 7-year-old with a broken elbow. I'm having a hard time feeling his pulse." The problems associated with managing distal humerus fractures in children are intimidating for any orthopedist. Attention to several key points facilitates the evaluation and management of this common pediatric elbow injury.

Pediatric supracondylar humerus fracture can occur in children and young teenagers; however, it is an injury seen most commonly between ages 5 and 8 years. Injuries to the left arm are more common than to the right. Girls are affected as frequently as boys. Concurrent fractures in the same limb are possible, particularly fractures of the forearm and distal radius.

## Relevant anatomy

Vascular insufficiency with a supracondylar fracture occurs in approximately 10% of children, and results from the proximity of the humerus to the brachial artery. The brachial artery passes along the anteromedial aspect of the humerus superficial to the brachialis. An extensive arborization of collateral arteries emanates from the vessel as it passes the anterior to the distal humerus. As the artery crosses the elbow it passes beneath the fascial extension of the biceps tendon, the lacertus fibrosis. In the proximal forearm, the artery splits into the radial and ulnar artery. The combination of the restraint of the lacertus fibrosis and the branching of the radial and ulnar artery fixes the artery distally. The proximal fragment of the fractured distal humerus can be driven through or around the brachialis and up against the brachial artery. The damaged artery appears abraded over several centimeters, suggesting that the bone has scraped along the effected length of the vessel. This results in intimal damage to the vessel that may lead to thrombosis. Complete occlusion of the brachial artery rarely leads to ischemia of the arm owing to the extensive collateral circulation about the elbow.

Nerve dysfunction has been reported in approximately 50% of children who have supracondylar humerus fractures. The median nerve crosses the elbow with the brachial artery. Posterolateral displacement of the fractured distal fragment results in anteromedial displacement of the proximal fragment. The proximal fragment is driven against the brachialis and the median nerve, a situation that can result in complete or more commonly partial median nerve neuropathy. The anterior interosseous nerve contusion is the most common form of post-traumatic neuropathy, constituting approximately 50% of all nerve injuries with pediatric supracondylar humerus fractures [1]. The radial nerve emerges from between the brachialis and brachioradialis muscles, crosses the elbow, and then penetrates the supinator muscle. Posteromedial displacement of the distal fragment means that the proximal fragment of the distal humerus is driven anterior and laterally toward the radial nerve. Radial nerve injuries account for approximately 30% of nerve injuries seen with supracondylar humerus fractures [1]. The ulnar nerve crosses the elbow posterior to the medial epicondyle as it passes through the cubital tunnel. A direct blow to the posterior aspect of the elbow as would be seen with a flexion-type supracondylar fracture can result in an ulnar nerve neurapraxia.

* Corresponding author.
*E-mail address:* mbaratz@wpahs.org (M. Baratz).

0749-0712/06/$ - see front matter © 2006 Elsevier Inc. All rights reserved.
doi:10.1016/j.hcl.2005.11.002

## Injury

Fall on an extended arm can impart a hyperextension moment to the elbow, particularly in children who have ligament laxity. The olecranon is driven into the olecranon fossa where a fracture is initiated. The fracture may be nondisplaced (type I), it may hinge on the posterior periosteum (type II) (Fig. 1), or the proximal fragment may displace and rotate tearing through adjacent soft tissues (type III) (Fig. 2). Hyperextension-type injuries account for approximately 90% of supracondylar fractures. Fall on the apex of the elbow can result in a flexion-type supracondylar fracture (10%).

## Diagnosis

The examiner needs to be sure the child did not injure the head or neck. Work around the elbow checking the shoulder, arm, forearm, wrist, and hand. The elbow will be swollen. In a displaced, type III fracture the proximal fragment is driven anteriorly. This may create an area of ecchymosis around the antecubital fossa. Carefully inspect this area for evidence of a skin break. Anterior displacement of the proximal fragment can result in injury to the brachial artery, median nerve, and radial nerve. Ecchymosis over the anteromedial aspect of the forearm is seen in association with brachial artery injuries (Fig. 3). The most common nerve injury is a partial median nerve neurapraxia involving the anterior interosseous portion of the median nerve [1]. This produces weakness of the flexor pollicis longus or the flexor digitorum profundus to the index finger, as evidenced by the inability to make the OK sign (Fig. 4).

Perfusion of the limb is assessed by evaluating color, capillary refill, and pulses. Loss of pulse should be confirmed with Doppler. Perfusion may improve following reduction of the fracture. An arteriogram of the limb may be indicated in the rare instance of persistent ischemia following fracture reduction and stabilization.

Radiographs of the entire limb should be taken, including the ipsilateral shoulder and wrist. No radiographs should be taken until the elbow is splinted in approximately 30° of flexion. Comparison views of the unaffected elbow can be helpful in subtle injuries and in younger children. Similarly an arthrogram, magnetic resonance (MR) imaging, or MR arthrograms can be used in those instances in which an injury is suspected but cannot be identified on plain radiographs.

There are several parameters that can be used to assess displacement and the quality of the fracture reduction. Three parameters are evaluated on an anteroposterior (AP) view. The outline of the olecranon fossa should appear circular.

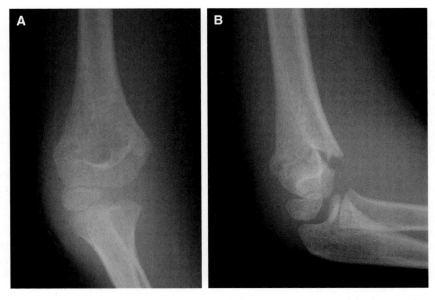

Fig. 1. (*A*) Anteroposterior (AP) view of a 7-year-old child who had a type II supracondylar humerus fracture. (*B*) Lateral view of a 7-year-old child who had a type II supracondylar humerus fracture.

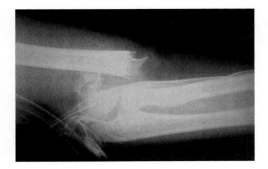

Fig. 2. Lateral view of a widely displaced type III supracondylar humerus fracture.

A line drawn down the axis of humerus should intersect with a line drawn along the lateral condylar physis at an angle of approximately 20° (Fig. 5). This is referred to as Baumann's Angle [2]. The medial epicondylar epiphyseal angle describes a line down the axis of humerus that intersects with a line along the medial epicondylar physis [3]. On a lateral view of the humerus a line drawn down the anterior cortex should bisect the capitellum. A line drawn down the axis of the humerus should form an angle of approximately 30° when it intersects with a line drawn through the center of the capitellum (Fig. 6).

## Treatment

The treating surgeon should strive for an anatomic reduction with immobilization in a position that does not place the child at risk for compartment syndrome. The following are pearls

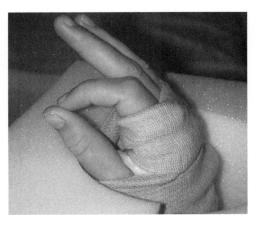

Fig. 4. Child who had a partial anterior interosseous nerve palsy (loss of flexor pollicus longus flexion).

to treatment that will ensure a satisfactory outcome (Box 1).

### Type I (nondisplaced)

A reduction maneuver is not necessary. The elbow is splinted in 90° flexion and neutral forearm rotation. Repeat radiographs are obtained at 1 week. A cast is applied and maintained until there is no tenderness over the distal humerus and there is radiographic evidence of healing. This usually takes 3 to 4 weeks.

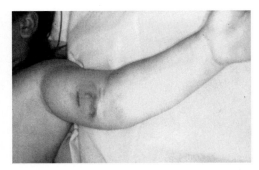

Fig. 3. Extensive ecchymosis over the anteromedial aspect of the elbow and forearm in a child who had a type III supracondylar humerus fracture and disruption of the brachial artery.

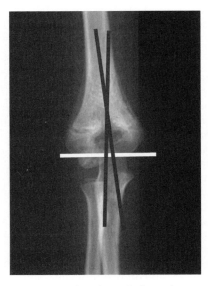

Fig. 5. Anteroposterior view of elbow demonstrating Baumann's angle.

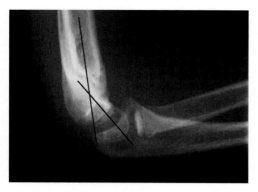

Fig. 6. Lateral view of elbow demonstrating the 30° angle that normally exists between the axis of the humeral shaft and the axis of the capitellum.

## Type II (angulated but not displaced, intact posterior periosteal hinge)

Most pediatric orthopedists now recommend closed reduction and percutaneous pin fixation (CRIF). Closed reduction and pinning ensures optimum reduction. Although extension is the primary deformity there may be an element of rotation that can be addressed concurrently. Closed reduction and pinning also eliminates the need to splint a swollen elbow in flexion, a position that potentially increases compartment pressures in the anterior compartment of the forearm. The posterior hinge of periosteum enhances stability of the reduced fracture. Two pins inserted through

---

**Box 1. Pearls**

Pearl: Unsure about displacement
  or quality of reduction? Get view
  of opposite elbow.
Pearl: Open reduction for open fractures,
  irreducible fractures, and fractures
  with ischemic hand.
Pearl: If one doesn't feel crepitus
  from the fracture and can't reduce
  the fracture, there may be interposed
  muscle, capsule, vessel, or nerve;
  open reduction by way of a transverse
  anterior incision with proximal
  extension up the medial side.
Pearl: Beware of the ulnar nerve. Expose
  medial epicondyle to ensure safe
  placement of a medial pin.

---

the lateral condyle provide the necessary stability. The authors believe the younger patient (6–8 years of age) who has minimal swelling and displacement can do well with closed reduction and a splint. This sentiment is supported by the work of Parikh and colleagues who found that 72% of children treated with closed reduction of a type II fracture maintained alignment throughout treatment [4]. As with any pediatric fracture, closed treatment requires close observation.

## Type III (100% displaced)

Completely displaced supracondylar fractures require reduction and percutaneous pin fixation. Under a general anesthetic the child is placed in a supine position on the operating table. A fluoroscopy unit is draped and the image intensifier is used as the arm board (Fig. 7). Longitudinal traction is applied to the arm with the forearm supinated. Medial–lateral translation of the distal fragment is corrected and verified with a posteroanterior (PA) projection. Rotation is corrected until the width of the metaphysis matches the width of the epiphysis on a PA image. For fractures with posteromedial displacement, flex the elbow and pronate the forearm while applying pressure on the tip of the olecranon with one's opposite thumb. Fractures with posterolateral displacement are reduced with flexion and forearm supination, and flexion-type injuries with elbow extension. The apices of the lateral epicondyle, olecranon, and medial epicondyle form an isosceles triangle in a normal, flexed elbow (Fig. 8). This relationship can be used to assess the quality of the fracture reduction. A PA image should be taken while maintaining the flexed and pronated position (Fig. 9). Interpretation can be

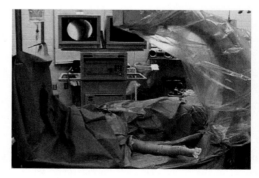

Fig. 7. C-arm draped for use in reducing and stabilizing a supracondylar humerus fracture.

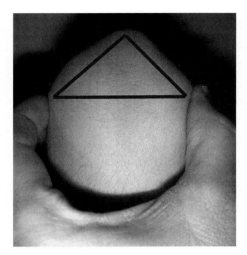

Fig. 8. Triangle formed on the posterior aspect of the flexed elbow caused by the normal relationship of the medial epicondyle, tip of the olecranon processes, and the lateral epicondyle.

more challenging because of the superimposed image of the forearm on the distal humerus. A lateral projection of the elbow is checked by externally rotating the shoulder while maintaining the flexed position of the elbow.

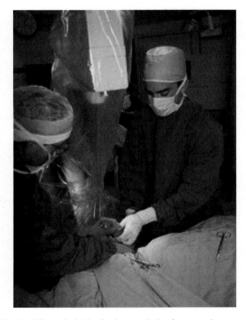

Fig. 9. Elbow held in flexion and the forearm in pronation to maintain the reduction of a type III supracondylar humerus fracture.

With the elbow still flexed, the tip of a 0.062-in pin is placed by hand against the lateral epicondyle and directed obliquely toward the medial metaphysis. The presumptive starting point and the planned angle of insertion are confirmed on PA fluoroscopic image. Advance the pin 2 cm into the bone and recheck the fracture reduction and pin position on a PA and a lateral projection. Advance the pin until it engages but does not penetrate fully the medial metaphyseal cortex. Recheck pin position and fracture reduction with intraoperative fluoroscopy. Place a second 0.062-in pin parallel to the first pin. The elbow is extended and radiographs are repeated. All type II and most type III fractures are sufficiently stable following placement of two lateral pins (Fig. 10). Placement of a third medial pin should be considered for type III fractures with metaphyseal comminution and extensive soft-tissue stripping. The authors recommend a small incision over the medial epicondyle to ensure safe placement of the medial pin [5].

*Open reduction*

Open reduction should be considered for fractures that have a skin break, an ischemic arm, or those that are irreducible. A small, anterior, J-shaped incision is made with the horizontal limb across the antecubital fossa and the vertical limb up the medial aspect of the arm. This approach allows the surgeon to evaluate the brachial artery and median nerve and to remove interposed soft tissue (Fig. 11). Open reduction through an anterior approach does not create an unsightly scar or limit motion [6]. With open reduction, the authors recommend placing one medial and two lateral pins.

*Vascular insufficiency*

The vascular status of the limb must be assessed when the child is first seen, again after manipulation of the fracture, and again following reduction with splint or reduction with pinning. A child who has a white, pulseless hand that does not pink up with fracture reduction should undergo brachial artery exploration and reconstruction. If the radial pulse is absent by palpation but present by Doppler or if the hand has capillary refill that is symmetric with the contralateral hand, observation is recommended. If there is no pulse by Doppler and the capillary refill is asymmetric, the authors recommend exploration

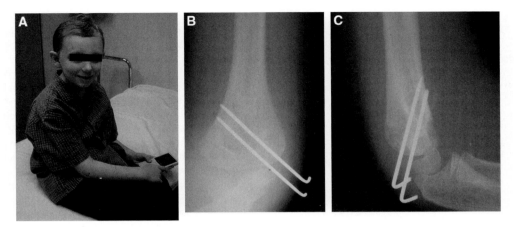

Fig. 10. (*A*) Two percutaneous placed pins in the lateral aspect of the elbow. (*B*) AP view of the elbow with two laterally placed pins. (*C*) Lateral view of the elbow with two laterally placed pins.

and reconstruction of the brachial artery. The authors also recommend admitting to the hospital any child in whom the vascular status is in question. Volkmann's ischemic contracture has become rare, because cast immobilization alone rarely is used to treat displaced supracondylar fractures. Surgeons must still be vigilant and decompress forearm compartments if compartment syndrome is suspected.

*Nerve deficits*

Most nerve deficits associated with supracondylar humerus fractures are neurapraxic injuries that resolve with observation. The exception is the deficit that becomes worse following fracture reduction. There are reports of the median nerve

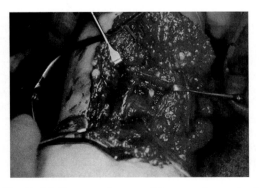

Fig. 11. Median nerve interposed between the proximal and distal ends of a widely displaced type III supracondylar humerus fracture.

becoming incarcerated in the fracture and of ulnar nerve injuries with percutaneous pin fixation [1,7]. In these instances, the nerve should be explored. Similarly, exploration should be considered for nerve deficits that persist beyond 3 months [1,7].

*Associated fractures*

Fractures of the forearm or distal radius can be seen concurrently with supracondylar humerus fractures. Roposch and colleagues reported that angulation of an associated forearm fracture occurred less frequently when the forearm fracture was treated with percutaneous pinning as compared with closed reduction and immobilization [8]. The combination of supracondylar and forearm fractures increases the possibility of compartment syndrome.

*Postoperative care*

Fractures treated with reduction and pin fixation are splinted in approximately 60° of flexion. In most cases the child is admitted and followed with examination of pulses, nerve function, and forearm compartments. The elbow is maintained in a splint for 3 to 4 weeks. Pins are removed when the distal humerus is no longer tender, usually in 3 to 4 weeks. The child is placed in a sling, which he or she subsequently forgets to wear, usually a day or two later.

*Therapy*

Keppler and colleagues studied two groups of children who had supracondylar humeral fractures without associated neurovascular deficits.

All children were treated by open reduction and internal fixation. Follow-up at 12 and 18 weeks showed better elbow motion in the children who underwent weekly therapy, but there was no difference in elbow motion after 1 year [9]. The authors do not recommend therapy unless the child has a persistent contracture after 3 to 4 months or has a persistent nerve deficit.

## Malunion

Cubitus varus has a reported incidence as high as 58% in type III fractures. Varus deformities are caused by rotational malalignment with or without medial physeal arrest [10]. Most varus deformities are cosmetic. Osteotomy with or without lateral epiphysiodesis is an option. Labele, however, reported a 33% complication with osteotomy of malunited supracondylar humerus fractures [11].

## Outcome

There is little information in the literature on the long-term function of children who were treated for a supracondylar fracture of the humerus. This is because most children do extremely well following appropriate treatment. In a prospective study of 116 fractures, Mazda and colleagues reported an excellent outcome in 99 (91.6%) children, a good outcome in 5 (4.6%), and a poor outcome in 4 (3.7%) [12]. The poor results were ascribed to technical errors in reduction that led to an unsatisfactory cosmetic result but good function. An excellent outcome is possible by adhering to the following principles:

1. Correct rotational and angular malalignment of the fracture
2. Pin fractures that are displaced or angulated, particularly in a swollen elbow so that the elbow can be immobilized in 50° to 60° of flexion
3. Check the status of vessels, nerves, and compartments before and after fracture treatment
4. If the fracture is irreducible, if nerve or vessel function is in question, open reduction through an anterior J-shaped incision allows

visualization of the median and ulnar nerve, the brachial artery, and the fracture

## References

[1] Campbell CC, Waters PM, Emans JB, et al. Neurovascular injury and displacement in type III supracondylar humerus fractures. J Pediatr Orthop 1995; 15:47–52.

[2] Camp J, Ishizue K, Gomez M, et al. Alteration of Baumann's angle by humeral position: implications for treatment of supracondylar humerus fractures. J Pediatr Orthop 1993;13:521–5.

[3] Biyani A, Gupta SP, Sharma JC. Determination of medial epicondylar epiphyseal angle for supracondylar humeral fractures in children. J Pediatr Orthop 1993;13:94–7.

[4] Royce RO, Dutkowsky JP, Kasser JR, et al. Neurologic complications after K-wire fixation of supracondylar humerus fractures in children. J Pediatr Orthop 1991;11:191–4.

[5] Labelle H, Bunnelll WP, Duhaime M, et al. Cubitus varus deformity following supracondylar fractures of the humerus in children. J Pediatr Orthop 1982; 2:539–46.

[6] Voss FR, Kasser JR, Trepman E, et al. Uniplanar supracondylar humeral osteotomy with preset Kirschner wires for posttraumatic cubitus varus. J Pediatr Orthop 1994;14:471–8.

[7] Keppler P, Salem K, Schwarting B, et al. The effectiveness of physiotherapy after operative treatment of supracondylar humeral fractures in children. J Pediatr Orthop 2005;25(3):314–6.

[8] Gosens T, Bongers KJ. Neurovascular complications and functional outcome in displaced supracondylar fractures of the humerus in children. Injury 2003;34(4):267–73.

[9] Parikh SN, Wall EJ, Foad S, et al. Displaced type II extension supracondylar humerus fractures—do they all need pinning? J Pediatr Orthop 2004;24.

[10] Mazda K, Boggione C, Fitoussi F, et al. Systematic pinning of displaced extension-type supracondylar fractures of the humerus in children. J Bone Joint Surg [Br] 2001;83-B:888–93.

[11] Ay S, Akinci M, Kamiloglu S, et al. Open reduction of displaced pediatric supracondylar humeral fractures through the anterior cubital approach. J Pediatr Orthop 2005;25(2):149–53.

[12] Roposch A, Reis M, Molina M, et al. Supracondylar fractures of the humerus associated with ipsilateral forearm fractures in children: a report of forty-seven cases. J Pediatr Orthop 2001;21(3):307–12.

# Pediatric Humeral Condyle Fractures

## Gloria R. Gogola, MD

*Department of Orthopaedics, University of Texas Health Science Center–Houston,
Houston, TX 77030, USA*

Distal humeral physeal fractures are common, accounting for 25% of pediatric elbow fractures. They are complex injuries involving an open physis and an articular surface. The fragments are mostly cartilaginous, making radiographic assessment difficult. Accurate diagnosis and prompt treatment are important to prevent complications and subsequent deformity.

## Fractures of the lateral condyle

Lateral condyle fractures account for 15% of all pediatric elbow fractures, making them the second most common elbow fracture in children [1]. Most occur between 4 and 10 years of age, with a peak incidence at 5 to 6 years [2]. The mechanism of injury is typically a varus force during a fall on a supinated forearm, with avulsion of the condylar fragment by the common extensor origin [1]. A less common mechanism is a compression injury from a fall on the palm with the elbow flexed, in which the radial head is driven into the lateral condyle [3].

Radiographic diagnosis is challenging, because a significant portion of the fragment is cartilaginous, especially in children younger than 5 years of age. A minimum of three views should be obtained, including an internal oblique view of the distal humerus [1]. Comparison views of the opposite elbow are helpful and should be obtained routinely. The exact location of a fracture line and the extent of displacement are hard to determine on plain radiographs and are often underestimated [4]. Varus and valgus stress views help determine stability of the fracture fragment; however, they are painful to perform and require heavy sedation.

*E-mail address:* Gloria.Gogola@uth.tmc.edu

Arthrography has been a useful adjunct to help delineate distal humerus physeal fractures. Yates and Sullivan noted the original diagnosis and treatment plan was altered in almost 20% of patients after arthrography, and that the injury pattern diagnosed most often was lateral condyle fractures [5]. Arthrography has a 92% sensitivity rate for detecting intra-articular extension, but false negatives can result if a hematoma blocks dye migration into the fracture line [6]. Additionally, it is a painful and invasive procedure, which limits its routine use. The most effective use of arthrography may be for intraoperative assessment of fracture reduction after closed reduction and pinning [7]. Other imaging modalities show promise in evaluating these difficult fractures, primarily MRI and ultrasound [8,9].

The Milch classification of lateral condyle fractures published in 1964 is perhaps the most well known. Milch described two basic fracture patterns. In type 1, which is rare, the fracture line passes through the secondary ossification center of the capitellum, exiting lateral to the capitellar–trochlear groove. Although the fragment may displace, the trochlea remains intact, providing inherent elbow stability. In type II, which is more common, the fracture line passes medial to the trochlear groove. There is potential elbow instability, because the radius and ulna can displace laterally with the fragment [1,10].

Mirsky and colleagues showed poor correlation between the preoperative radiographic diagnosis and intraoperative findings using the Milch classification [11]. There is a shift in the literature toward classifying these fractures based on amount of displacement. Type I fractures are displaced less than 2 mm, type II fractures are 2 to 4 mm displaced, and type III fractures (Fig. 1) are completely displaced and rotated [12].

0749-0712/06/$ - see front matter © 2006 Elsevier Inc. All rights reserved.
doi:10.1016/j.hcl.2005.09.003

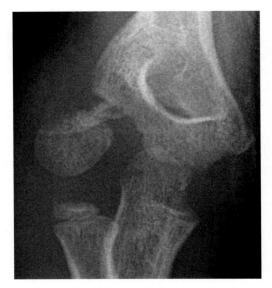

Fig. 1. AP radiograph of a type III lateral condyle fracture. (Courtesy of Howard R. Epps, MD, Houston, TX.)

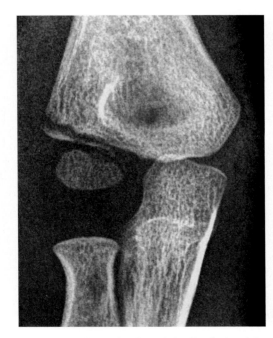

Fig. 2. AP radiograph of a minimally displaced but complete lateral condyle fracture. (Courtesy of Howard R. Epps, MD, Houston, TX.)

The treatment of type I (non- or minimally displaced) fractures is controversial. They are considered stable fractures, but it is well recognized that they can displace over time [13,14]. Although most displace within 5 to 7 days of injury [15,16], late displacement leading to nonunion can occur in 5% to 10% of cases [17]. The current recommendation is to treat up to 2 mm displacement nonoperatively with close follow-up, including serial radiographs out of plaster [16,18,19]. Healing of the lateral condyle can take longer than other elbow fractures, and many investigators have noted that 6 to 12 weeks of immobilization may be required for successful closed treatment [14,20,21].

It is useful to identify accurately the subset of these stable fractures most likely to displace and treat them more aggressively. Jakob and colleagues noted that type I fractures can be complete or incomplete [12]. In incomplete fractures, the fracture line stops before passing through the entire cartilaginous epiphysis, leaving a cartilaginous hinge that makes the fragment stable and therefore unlikely to displace. Conversely if the hinge is disrupted, there is a complete fracture that exits into the joint (Fig. 2). The strong extensor muscle group attached to the fragment then can exert a deforming force, rotating and displacing the condyle. A complete fracture should be considered unstable and at risk for further displacement, despite an initial radiograph showing less than 2 mm of displacement.

Clearly visualizing fracture line propagation through an unossified trochlear region with plain radiographs is often difficult and sometimes not possible. MRI has been shown to visualize reliably the area in question. Horn and colleagues recently correlated MRI and radiographs to clinical course to determine fracture stability [8]. The study followed 16 children, 2 to 8 years of age, all of whom healed without complication in an average of 5.5 weeks. The clearly unstable fractures on plain radiographs (greater than 3 mm initial displacement) were treated surgically. The radiographically stable fractures with an intact cartilaginous hinge on MRI were treated in casts; none subsequently displaced. There were two fractures initially classified as stable by radiographs and treated in casts that were actually complete on MRI. Of these, one displaced within the first week and was treated surgically. MRI scans are still expensive and require sedation in young children, and so should not be used routinely in all fractures. It is a useful tool, however, in evaluating fractures in which plain radiographs are not clear and fracture stability is in question.

Complete fractures, even though initially nondisplaced, can be treated more aggressively with percutaneous pinning to avoid displacement and the risk for nonunion [4].

The treatment of type II fractures (2–4 mm displacement) is evolving. Previously, open reduction, internal fixation (ORIF) was recommended for all fractures with greater than 2 mm initial displacement; closed reduction and percutaneous pinning represents a newer trend. Even up to 3 to 4 mm of displacement can be treated by closed reduction and pinning as long as anatomic reduction is achieved [19,22,23]. Reduction is best confirmed by intraoperative arthrography [19]. Rotation of the fracture fragment is difficult to reduce with closed techniques and may require open reduction. Closed reduction, under anesthesia and with fluoroscopic guidance, is performed with the elbow flexed and the forearm supinated. A smooth K-wire can be used percutaneously as a joystick. Fixation is achieved with two smooth K-wires across the physis or with a cannulated screw across the metaphysis if the metaphyseal spike is of sufficient size. An evidence-based comparison of closed reduction and percutaneous pinning with arthrogram versus ORIF showed no significant difference between the two techniques [24].

There is consensus that unstable type II and all type III fractures require ORIF [13,14,18] (Fig. 3). As early as 1933 these were deemed a fracture of necessity for surgical stabilization [25]. A lateral approach is used through the interval between the brachioradialis and triceps. It is important to minimize dissection of the fragment during reduction, particularly the posterior aspect where the blood supply originates. Fragment fixation is achieved with two smooth K-wires through the epiphysis or the metaphyseal spike, or if the fragment is large enough, with screw fixation through the metaphysis [4] (Fig. 4A,B).

Catgut suture fixation has been used previously but provides inadequate strength to maintain fixation [22]. Biodegradable fixation, in the form of rods and screws, has been reported in children with results equal to metal pins [26,27]. There are no long-term results published yet in these small studies, however, and the effect of biodegradable materials on open physes has not been shown definitively. Postoperatively, the elbow is immobilized in a posterior long arm splint at 90° flexion. The K-wires are removed when there is evidence of radiographic healing, usually 6 weeks [28], although a recent study suggests that 3 weeks may be sufficient [29].

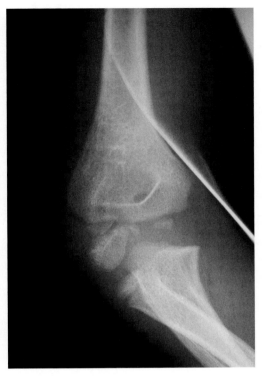

Fig. 3. AP radiographs of a 6-year-old boy with displaced lateral condyle fracture secondary to a fall. (Courtesy of Shriners Hospital for Children, Philadelphia, PA.)

Lateral condyle fractures are one of a few pediatric fractures in which nonunion is a common complication [4]. In a review of 53 fractures, Beaty and Wood noted that all of the fractures treated with ORIF healed. Of those treated closed, they found a 28.5% nonunion rate. Long-term follow-up of a subset of initially unrecognized, untreated fractures that went on to nonunion showed further complications, including cubitus valgus deformity, weakness, loss of elbow motion, occasional pain, and tardy ulnar nerve palsy [4]. Another long-term study suggests that nonunion symptoms correlate with the original fracture type. Eighteen patients with 19 fractures were reviewed. The average age was 5.4 years (range, 3–10 years) at injury and 42.5 years (range, 20–78 years) at follow-up. Original Milch type I fracture types consistently had pain, instability, loss of motion, and ulnar nerve dysfunction. In the Milch type II fractures, disabling symptoms were rare; this group occasionally showed clinically detectable ulnar nerve symptoms. The study

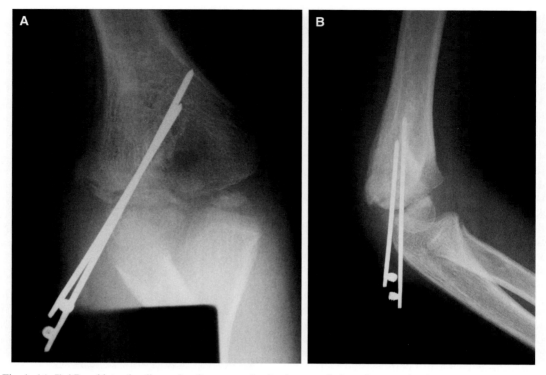

Fig. 4. (*A*, *B*) AP and lateral radiographs after open reduction by way of a lateral approach using two smooth Kirschner wires. (Courtesy of Shriners Hospital for Children, Philadelphia, PA.)

investigators recommended treating Milch type I nonunions as soon as possible, preferably before skeletal maturity [30].

Nonunions are at risk for progressive displacement, with the fragment migrating proximally, increasing valgus deformity and developing tardy ulnar nerve palsy [1,13,31,32]. Most investigators therefore currently advocate prompt surgical treatment of a nonunion once it is recognized. Treatment is guided by the amount of displacement and timing of diagnosis. Up to 4 to 5 mm of displacement can be anatomically reduced and pinned up to 6 weeks postinjury with good results [33]. If a nonunion is recognized early (before 12 weeks from injury) and is minimally displaced, it should be fixed in situ. A minimally invasive technique is used, such as percutaneous pins, or if age appropriate, cannulated screws for compression [19]. Once a nonunion is more than 12 weeks from injury, attempted reduction is not advocated because of the risk for avascular necrosis (AVN). At that point an open approach with bone grafting and internal fixation generally is needed [14,34]. The goal is to achieve bony union

to prevent valgus deformity and subsequent ulnar nerve problems and to relieve pain; some loss of motion should be expected [34].

The cubitus valgus deformity of an established nonunion results from the proximal migration of the lateral condyle fragment, not from premature closure of the capitellar physis [4]. There are two surgical approaches to treat this difficult problem: a one-stage intra-articular osteotomy and a staged approach with an extra-articular osteotomy for deformity correction. In the former, an intra-articular osteotomy with partial reduction and bone grafting is performed. The goal is to fix the fragment in a position of best functional range of motion, not anatomic restoration [33]. The common extensor origin can be lengthened to assist in reduction [35]. In a staged approach, the lateral condyle is bone grafted and fixed in situ and the ulnar nerve transposed. When bone healing has occurred and motion returned, a supracondylar corrective osteotomy is performed as second stage [19].

Another complication of lateral condyle fractures is premature closure of the central portion of the physis, resulting in what is referred to commonly as a fishtail deformity (Fig. 5A,B). The term, coined in 1955, describes the inverted U or V shape resulting from the continued growth of the medial and lateral portions of the physis. It has been attributed to incomplete reduction, AVN, and central physeal bar formation [36]. Length discrepancy is seen rarely, because the distal humerus contributes little (15%–20%) to the overall longitudinal growth of the humerus [1]. It is a deformity that is generally well tolerated in children, hence there is not much written about it in the literature. Recently there has been some concern over problems developing later in adulthood, including premature degenerative arthrosis, deformity, disability, and possible higher risk for intercondylar fracture. There is no primary treatment for AVN of the distal humeral epiphysis and no reports of physeal bar excision. Once partial physeal arrest is noted, however, future deformity could be minimized by surgical arrest of the remainder of the physis, with little to no functional length discrepancy expected [36].

## Fractures of the medial condyle

Medial condyle fractures account for less than 2% of all pediatric elbow fractures, typically seen between 8 and 12 years of age [3,37,38]. They represent a Salter-Harris IV physeal injury. There are two mechanisms of injury similar to the lateral condyle fractures. One is an avulsion by the flexor–pronator mass from valgus stress in a fall on an outstretched arm; the second is a compression injury from a fall on a flexed elbow in which the olecranon is driven into the medial condyle [39]. Associated ulnar nerve injury is extremely rare [38].

Diagnosis is difficult, because these fractures commonly occur before the trochlea has ossified. They often are mistaken for medial epicondylar fractures, leading to a delay in care and poor outcome [38]. The risk for misdiagnosis is highest in younger children. A suspected medial epicondyle fracture in a young child whose trochlea has not yet ossified should be examined under varus and valgus stress. Epicondyle fractures are associated with elbow dislocations and valgus instability, whereas condyle fractures are unstable in varus because of injury to the medial column [39]. Arthrography and MRI may be useful, but ultimately a high index of suspicion is required.

Medial condyle fractures are classified much like lateral condyle fractures [40]. Type I is a greenstick or impacted fracture, type II is a complete fracture with intra-articular extension but

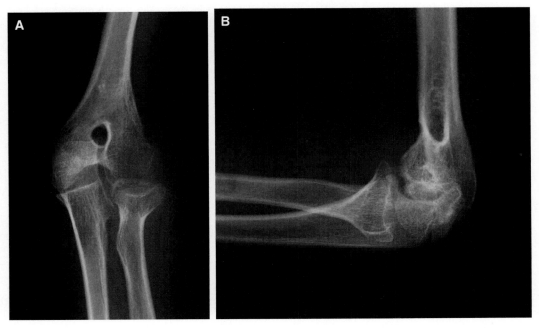

Fig. 5. (*A, B*) A 12-year-old girl with a previous lateral condyle fracture. AP and lateral radiographs reveal a fishtail deformity. (Courtesy of Shriners Hospital for Children, Philadelphia, PA.)

minimal articular gap, and type III is a displaced and rotated fragment. The deforming force is the forearm flexor–pronator mass [39].

Type I and nondisplaced type II fractures are treated with cast immobilization with the elbow in flexion and neutral rotation. ORIF is recommended for displacement greater than 2 mm [41]. Potential complications include nonunion, physeal injury, AVN, cubitus varus deformity, and loss of elbow motion.

### Medial epicondyle fractures

Medial epicondyle fractures account for approximately 10% of pediatric elbow fractures. The peak incidence is 10 to 14 years of age, and 75% are seen in boys [22]. The mechanism of injury is typically an avulsion of the epicondylar apophysis by the forearm flexors when a valgus load is applied to the elbow in a fall on the outstretched arm [4]. Up to 50% occur with posterior–lateral elbow dislocation [42].

Classification of medial epicondylar fractures is based on the degree of displacement (more or less than 5 mm), whether or not the fragment is incarcerated in the joint, and the presence or absence of concomitant dislocation [43].

Fractures with less than 5 mm displacement do well with immobilization at 90° of flexion for 5 to 7 days (Fig. 6A,B). Protected elbow motion then is begun to prevent stiffness [44,45]. Some advocate treating all medial epicondyle fractures closed, noting that nonunions are mostly asymptomatic or easily treated with excision of the fragment [46] (Fig. 7). Good results have been obtained with late extraction of incarcerated fragments, with return of 80% of normal motion [47].

If the epicondyle is visible on a lateral radiograph, it is likely trapped in the joint [48]. A closed maneuver may be attempted to free a trapped fragment. With the arm supinated and slightly flexed, a valgus stress is applied to the elbow joint. Passive extension of the fingers may help put traction on epiphysis [45]. Of note, there may be ulnar or median nerve entrapment in the joint also, so multiple vigorous attempts at closed reduction should be avoided.

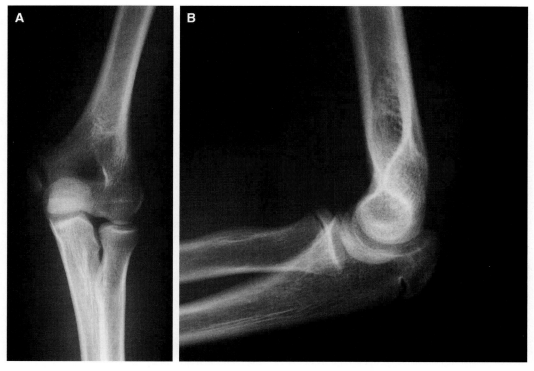

Fig. 6. (A, B) A 15-year-old wrestler injured during a match. AP and lateral radiographs reveal a minimally displaced medial epicondyle fracture. (Courtesy of Shriners Hospital for Children, Philadelphia, PA.)

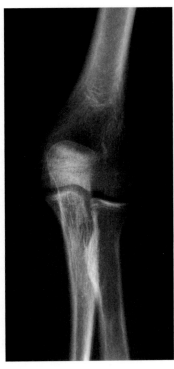

Fig. 7. Subsequent radiographs reveal union of the medial epicondyle fracture. (Courtesy of Shriners Hospital for Children, Philadelphia, PA.)

Absolute indications for ORIF are open fractures and irreducible dislocations or incarcerated fragments [3]. Relative indications are less defined. Although there is no consensus on a specific amount of displacement that requires open treatment, 2 to 5 mm are generally accepted values [3,49,50]. Less displacement or valgus instability is considered a surgical indication in the dominant arm of competitive gymnasts or throwing athletes [22,51]. Woods and Tullos showed that medial elbow stability depends on the three bands of the medial collateral ligament and the forearm flexors. When the medial epicondyle displaces, the entire collateral ligament displaces with it, losing its tightness and resulting in medial instability of the elbow [22]. Ulnar nerve symptoms were previously believed to be an indication for surgical exploration; however, studies have shown no permanent nerve injuries from this type of fracture. Observation is currently recommended [3,44]. Median nerve symptoms, although rare, are an indication for operative exploration [3].

Fixation can be achieved with smooth K-wires or a cannulated screw and must be stable enough to allow early motion. Elbow stiffness is the most common complication, especially with a concomitant dislocation [3]. An evolving alternative to open reduction is fluoroscopically-guided percutaneous fixation in conjunction with elbow arthroscopy, particularly in athletes [52].

## Lateral epicondyle fractures

Lateral epicondyle fractures are rare. They occur primarily in the second decade. Treatment is usually cast immobilization, followed by early motion when tolerated. Displacement greater than 5 mm can lead to joint stiffness; this can be treated with fragment excision [1,3].

## Osteochondral fractures of the capitellum

Capitellar fractures may be seen in adolescents older than 12 years, especially in athletes. The adult classification is used: type I is a large trochlear fragment, type II is an articular fragment with minimal subchondral bone, and type III is comminuted.

Treatment is fragment excision or internal fixation through an open approach or arthroscopically [3]. Operative reduction is usually successful in restoring functional elbow motion [53].

## Summary

Condylar and epicondylar fractures differ from other pediatric upper extremity fractures because of the anatomy and ossification of the distal humerus. These fractures are prone to nonunion, and initial deformities do not remodel well. Radiographic diagnosis and severity are difficult to determine, and adjunct studies, particularly arthrography and MRI, often are needed. The correlation of an intact cartilaginous hinge and subsequent fracture stability has helped identify fractures at risk for displacement and nonunion, prompting closer follow-up or more aggressive initial treatment. Although many humeral condylar fractures can be treated successfully with cast immobilization, operative treatment often is warranted. Specific treatment recommendations continue to evolve. The general trend is toward treating more fractures and nonunions with surgical fixation while using less invasive techniques.

## References

[1] Price C, Phillips J, Devito D. Management of fractures. In: Morrissy, Weinstein SL, editors. Lovell

& Winter's pediatric orthopaedics. 5th edition. Philadelphia: Lippincott Williams & Wilkins; 2001. p. 1319–422.

[2] dePablos J, Tejero A. Fractures of the upper limb and hand. In: Benson MK, Fixen JA, Macnicol MF, et al, editors. Children's orthopaedics and fractures. 2nd edition. New York: Churchill Livingston; 2002. p. 609–32.

[3] Green NE. Fractures and dislocations about the elbow. In: Green NE, Swiontkowski MF, editors. Skeletal trauma in children. 3rd edition. Philadelphia: WB Saunders; 2003. p. 257–321.

[4] Canale ST. Fractures and dislocations. In: Canale ST, Beaty JH, editors. Operative pediatric orthopaedics. 2nd edition. St. Louis: Mosby; 1995. p. 913–1111.

[5] Yates C, Sullivan JA. Arthrographic diagnosis of elbow injuries in children. J Pediatr Orthop 1987;7(1): 54–60.

[6] Marzo JM, d'Amato C, Strong M, et al. Usefulness and accuracy of arthrography in management of lateral humeral condyle fractures in children. J Pediatr Orthop 1990;10:317–21.

[7] Noonan KJ. Lateral condyle fracture nonunion. In: Price CT, editor. Complications in orthopaedics: pediatric upper extremity fractures. Rosemont (IL): American Academy of Orthopaedic Surgeons; 2004. p. 29–37.

[8] Horn BD, Herman MJ, Crisci K, et al. Fractures of the lateral humeral condyle: role of the cartilage hinge in fracture stability. J Pediatr Orthop 2002; 22:8–11.

[9] Vocke-Hell AK, Schmid A. Sonographic differentiation of stable and unstable lateral condyle fractures of the humerus in children. J Pediatr Orthop B 2001;10:138–41.

[10] Milch HJ. Fractures and fracture dislocations of the humeral condyles. J Trauma 1964;15:592–607.

[11] Mirsky EC, Karas EH, Weiner LS. Lateral condyle fractures in children: evaluation of classification and treatment. J Orthop Trauma 1997;11:117–20.

[12] Jakob R, Fowles JV, Rang M, et al. Observations concerning fractures of the lateral humeral condyle in children. J Bone Joint Surg [Br] 1975;57:430–6.

[13] Flynn JC. Nonunion of slightly displaced fractures of the lateral humeral condyle in children: an update. J Pediatr Orthop 1989;9:691–6.

[14] Flynn JC, Richards JF Jr, Saltzman RI. Prevention and treatment of nonunion of slightly displaced fractures of the lateral humeral condyle in children. An end-result study. J Bone Joint Surg 1975;57A: 1087–92.

[15] Pirker ME, Weinberg AM, Hollwarth ME, et al. Subsequent displacement of initially nondisplaced and minimally displaced fractures of the lateral humeral condyle in children. J Trauma 2005;58:1202–7.

[16] Finnbogason T, Karsson G, Lindberg L, et al. Nondisplaced and minimally displaced fractures of the lateral humeral condyle in children: a prospective radiographic investigation of fracture stability. J Pediatr Orthop 1995;15:422–5.

[17] Flynn JM, Sarwark JF, Waters PM, et al. The surgical management of pediatric fractures of the upper extremity. Instr Course Lect 2003;52:635–45.

[18] Badelon O, Bensahel H, Mazda K, et al. Lateral humeral condylar fractures in children: a report of 47 cases. J Pediatr Orthop 1988;8:31–4.

[19] Papandrea R, Waters P. Posttraumatic reconstruction of the elbow in the pediatric patient. Clin Orthop Rel Res 2000;370:115–26.

[20] Flynn JC, Richards JF. Non-union of minimally displaced fractures of the lateral condyle of the humerus in children. J Bone Joint Surg 1971;53A: 1096–101.

[21] Bast SC, Hoffer MM, Aval S. Non-operative treatment for minimally and non-displaced lateral humeral condyle fractures in children. J Pediatr Orthop 1998;18:448–50.

[22] Woods GW, Tullos HS. Elbow instability and medial epicondyle fractures. Am J Sports Med 1977;5: 23–30.

[23] Mintzer CM, Waters PM, Brown DJ, et al. Percutaneous pinning in the treatment of displaced lateral condyle fractures. J Pediatr Orthop 1994;14:462–5.

[24] Bhandari M, Tornetta P, Swiontkowski M. Displaced lateral condyle fractures of the distal humerus. J Pediatr Trauma 2003;17:306–8.

[25] Speed JS, Macey HB. Fractures of the humeral condyles in children. J Bone Joint Surg 1933;15:903–19.

[26] Svensson PJ, Janarv PM, Hirsch G. Internal fixation with biodegradable rods in pediatric fractures: one year follow up of fifty patients. J Pediatr Orthop 1994;14:220–4.

[27] Mäkelä EA, Böstman O, Kekomäki M, et al. Biodegradable fixation of distal humeral physeal fractures. Clin Orthop 1992;283:237–43.

[28] Cardona JI, Riddle E, Kumar SJ. Displaced fractures of the lateral humeral condyle: criteria for implant removal. J Pediatr Orthop 2002;22:194–7.

[29] Thomas DP, Howard AW, Cole WG, et al. Three weeks of Kirschner wire fixation for displaced lateral condylar fractures of the humerus in children. J Pediatr Orthop 2001;21:565–9.

[30] Toh S, Tsubo K, Nishikawa S, et al. Long-standing nonunion of fractures of the lateral humeral condyle. J Bone Joint Surg 2002;84A(4):593–8.

[31] DeBoeck H. Surgery for nonunion of the lateral humeral condyle in children. 6 cases followed for 1–9 years. Acta Orthop Scand 1995;66(5):401–2.

[32] Wilkins KE. Residuals of elbow trauma in children. Orthop Clin North Am 1990;21(2):291–314.

[33] Roye D, Bini S, Infosino A. Late surgical treatment of lateral condylar fractures in children. J Pediatr Orthop 1991;11:195–9.

[34] Masada K, Kawai H, Kawabata H, et al. Osteosynthesis for old, established nonunion of the lateral condyle of the humerus. J Bone Joint Surg 1990; 72A:32–40.

[35] Gaur SC, Varma AN, Swarup A. A new surgical technique for old ununited lateral condyle fractures of the humerus in children. J Trauma 1993;34:68–9.

[36] Nwakama AC, Peterson HA, Shaughnessy WJ. Fishtail deformity following fracture of the distal humerus in children: historical review, case presentations, discussion of etiology, and thoughts on treatment. J Pediatr Orthop B 2000;9(4): 309–18.

[37] Bensahel H, Csukonyi Z, Badelon O, et al. Fractures of the medial condyle of the humerus in children. J Pediatr Orthop 1986;6:430–3.

[38] Leet AI, Young C, Hoffer MM. Medial condyle fractures of the humerus in children. J Pediatr Orthop 2002;22:2–7.

[39] Goodwin RC, Kuivila TE. Pediatric elbow and forearm fractures requiring surgical treatment. Hand Clin 2002;18:135–48.

[40] Kilfoyle RM. Fractures of the medial condyle and epicondyle in children. Clin Orthop Rel Res 1965; 41:43–50.

[41] Papavasiliou V, Nenopoulos S, Venturis T. Fractures of the medial condyle of the humerus in childhood. J Pediatr Orthop 1987;7:421–3.

[42] Fowles JV, Slimane N, Kassab MT. Elbow dislocation with avulsion of the medial humeral epicondyle. J Bone Joint Surg [Br] 1990;72:102–4.

[43] Smith FM. Children's elbow injuries: fractures and dislocations. Clin Orthop Rel Res 1967;50:7–30.

[44] Bernstein SM, King JD, Sanderson RA. Fractures of the medial epicondyle of the humerus. Contemp Orthop 1981;12:637–41.

[45] Beaty JH. Elbow fractures in children and adolescents. Instr Course Lect 2003;52:661–5.

[46] Josefsson P, Danielsson J. Epicondylar elbow fracture in children. 35-year follow up of 56 unreduced cases. Acta Orthop Scand 1986;57:313–5.

[47] Fowles JV, Kassab MT, Muola T. Untreated intra-articular entrapment of the medial humeral epicondyle. J Bone Joint Surg [Br] 1984;60:562–5.

[48] Patrick J. Fracture of the medial epicondyle with displacement into the elbow joint. J Bone Joint Surg 1946;28:143–7.

[49] Duun PS, Ravn P, Hansen LB, et al. Osteosynthesis of medial humeral epicondyle fractures in children: 8-year follow-up of 33 cases. Acta Orthop Scand 1994;65(4):439–41.

[50] Hines RF, Herndon WA, Evans JP. Operative treatment of medial epicondyle fractures in children. Clin Orthop Rel Res 1987;223:170–4.

[51] Case SL, Hennrikus WL. Surgical treatment of displaced medial epicondyle fractures in adolescent athletes. Am J Sports Med 1997;25:682–6.

[52] Holt MS, Savoie FH 3rd, Field LD, et al. Arthroscopic management of elbow trauma. Hand Clin 2004;20:485–95.

[53] Letts M, Rumball K, Bauermeister S, et al. Fractures of the capitellum in adolescents. J Pediatr Orthop 1997;17:315–20.

ELSEVIER
SAUNDERS

Hand Clin 22 (2006) 87–98

HAND
CLINICS

# Nerve Palsies Related to Pediatric Upper Extremity Fractures

Harish S. Hosalkar, MD, MBMS (Orth)[a], Jonas L. Matzon, MD[a],
Benjamin Chang, MD, FACS[a,b],*

[a]*The Children's Hospital of Philadelphia, Division of Orthopedic Surgery, 2nd Floor, Wood Building,
34th Street and Civic Center Boulevard, Philadelphia, PA 19104, USA*
[b]*Division of Plastic Surgery, Hospital of the University of Pennsylvania, 10 Penn Tower, 3400 Spruce Street,
Philadelphia, PA 19104, USA*

Injuries to peripheral nerves are common in all forms of pediatric upper extremity trauma, including fractures, dislocations, ligamentous tears, and crush or amputation injuries. Common causes include falls and collisions, including athletic competitions, motor vehicle accidents, penetrating trauma, and occasionally industrial accidents. Approximately 80% to 90% of nerve injuries associated with fractures occur in the upper extremity [1]. Nerve injuries are associated with approximately 2.5% of extremity fractures in children and are more than twice as likely to be found with upper extremity fractures than with lower extremity fractures [2]. The incidence of neural injuries associated with specific injuries like supracondylar humeral fractures in children has been estimated to be 10% to 20% in most modern series [3,4], with a male preponderance noted of approximately 3:2 compared with girls [5,6]. The reported incidence of radial nerve injury is up to 16% with humeral fractures [7]. Noble and colleagues reported a trauma population of 5,777 patients (adults and children) treated between January 1, 1986 and November 30, 1996 in which 162 patients sustained 200 peripheral nerve injuries, 121 of which were in the upper extremity. The most frequently injured nerve was the radial nerve [8].

In the upper extremity, fractures that are associated with loss of nerve function present the treating physician with challenges beyond the primary initial goals of successful skeletal stabilization and soft-tissue coverage. Also, the recognition of peripheral nerve lesions may be more difficult in a polytrauma child, who may be obtunded, necessitating a thorough neurologic evaluation of all polytrauma patients, with follow-up electrodiagnostic evaluation as needed.

## Classification of nerve injuries

Injuries to peripheral nerves represent injury to axons and target-end organs. Nerve injury patterns may vary from fascicle to fascicle and along the longitudinal axis of the nerve. There are three main systems for classifying nerve injuries developed by Seddon in 1943, Sunderland in 1951, and Mackinnon in 1992 [9–11]. It is critical to understand these classifications for a clinician planning to manage these nerve injuries.

Seddon described three types of nerve injuries [9]: neuropraxia, axonotmesis, and neurotmesis. Sunderland expanded this to identify 2° of nerve injuries intermediate between axonotmesis and neurotmesis. Mackinnon added the concept of mixed injury or neuroma in continuity.

Neuropraxia (Sunderland first-degree injury) describes an injury with no disruption of the internal structure of the nerve. This usually involves

None of the authors have received any funding or support from any interested parties in the preparation of this manuscript.

* The Children's Hospital of Philadelphia, Department of Orthopedic Surgery, 2nd Floor, Wood Building, 34th Street and Civic Center Boulevard, Philadelphia, PA 19104.

*E-mail address:* Chang@email.chop.edu (B. Chang).

a localized area of conduction block. Tinel sign is not present, because there is no axonal abnormality. Loss of function initially may be complete, but there is no axonal degeneration and full recovery can be anticipated. Axonotmesis (Sunderland second-degree injury) represents injury to the axons such that Wallerian degeneration occurs distal to the level of the injury. Tinel sign progresses distally at the rate of 1 inch per month, corresponding to axonal regeneration. Surgical treatment generally is not required and close to normal function can be expected as the final outcome following the injury unless the level of injury is so far from the sensory or motor targets that time of denervation becomes a factor in influencing ultimate end organ function.

Sunderland's third- and fourth-degree injuries are included as extensions of axonotmesis and neurotmesis, respectively, in Seddon's classification. Sunderland's third-degree injury, in which the axonal injury is associated with endoneurial scarring, yields the most variable ultimate recovery. In Sunderland's fourth-degree injury the nerve is in continuity, but at the level of injury there is complete scarring across the nerve such that regeneration cannot occur. Tinel sign is usually present at the time of injury but does not proceed distally. Neurotmesis (or Sunderland fifth-degree injury) implies a complete transection of the nerve and interruption of continuity of all the neural tissues. There is no potential for spontaneous recovery. After repair, nerve regeneration can take place at the rate of approximately 1 mm per day, and return of some nerve function may be expected.

Mackinnon's mixed injury [11], or grade VI injury, combines various injury patterns from fascicle to fascicle and along the longitudinal length of the nerve. It provides the greatest surgical challenge in that normal fascicles or those with

potential for good recovery must be protected, while fascicles with Sunderland fourth- and fifth-degree injuries are reconstructed using repair or grafting techniques. The degree of injury, Tinel sign, recovery pattern, and rate for different nerve injuries are summarized in Table 1.

## Physiology of nerve transection

Following nerve transection, physiologic changes occur within the severed nerve end that are referred to as Wallerian degeneration [12]. In the distal part, Schwann cells and macrophages phagocytose the degenerating axons and myelin sheath. The endoneurial tube is preserved but progressively narrows in diameter over time. Proximally similar changes occur for a short distance [13]. At the cell body, the nucleus migrates from a central to a more peripheral position and increases in size. Cellular activity shifts from production of neurotransmitters to synthesis of membrane proteins. Some cells within the cell body do not survive, and the degree of cell death is related to the age of the patient and proximity of transection.

Peripheral nerve and end-organ changes occurring after nerve injury are of fundamental importance when considering management. In clinical practice, only extremity volume and circumference have been used to document changes following fractures with nerve injury. One month after denervation there is approximately 30% muscle atrophy; by 2 months 50% to 60%; and by 3 months 60% to 80%. After 3 months, equilibrium is reached and further detectable atrophy is minimal. Cross-sectional area diminishes 80% to 90% by 90 days [14]. Clinically the loss of function after varying periods of denervation can be estimated based on Woodhall and

Table 1
Physiology of nerve transection

|     | Degree of injury | Tinel sign present/ progresses distally | Recovery pattern | Rate of recovery | Surgical procedure |
|-----|------------------|------------------------------------------|------------------|------------------|---------------------|
| I   | Neuropraxia      | −/−                                      | Complete         | Fast, days to 12 weeks | None |
| II  | Axonotmesis      | +/+                                      | Complete         | Slow (1 in/month) | None |
| III | Axonotmesis      | +/+                                      | Variation        | Slow (1 in/month) | None or neurolysis |
| IV  | Axonotmesis      | +/−                                      | None             | No recovery       | Nerve repair or nerve graft |
| V   | Neurotmesis      | −/−                                      | None             | No recovery       | Nerve repair or nerve graft |
| VI  | Mixed, neuroma in continuity | Varies with each fascicle, depending on the combination of injury patterns | | | |

Beebe's determination that 1% function is lost for every 6 days of denervation [15].

## Diagnosis of nerve injury

Confirmation of a nerve injury is not usually difficult but can be tricky, especially in the pediatric population. If the nerve is completely transected, there is obvious immediate lack of active movement in the motor distribution of the nerve caused by paralysis of these muscles. In the upper extremity, each of the three major nerves (radial, median, and ulnar) should be assessed critically. Assessment of pinch, grip, and individual muscle function is recommended. When the motor disturbances are minimal or overshadowed by more striking sensory deficits, the injury may remain undiagnosed if a thorough examination is not performed on a coherent patient.

Sensory examination should be performed on a calm and sober patient who is blinded to the sensory examination. The two-point discrimination test must be done with the patient's eyes closed. This test reflects the innervation density and provides an indication of the number of innervated receptors. Static and moving two-point discrimination should be performed when possible. Vibrometer (a more sensitive test of receptor function) may be used to quantify the threshold of the quickly adapting fibers. Pressure thresholds can be assessed quantitatively using the Semmes-Weinstein monofilaments [11]. Sensibility examination, however, is difficult in young children. They often do not understand the term "numbness" or comprehend the test for sensation. These difficulties explain the frequent delayed presentation of nerve injury in children.

When there is a suspicion of a partial nerve injury, the examination must be detailed to reveal any motor or sensory deficit. The examination is more difficult with complex injuries involving muscle, tendon, and bone. Other neurologic injuries, intense pain, or intoxication also may alter the examination findings.

In addition to any sensory deficit in the cutaneous distribution of the nerve, a loss of ability to produce sweat coexists in the same area. This absence is established immediately after the injury but can be seen after a few days when the skin is dry, smooth, and polished. Laboratory examination with ninhydrin that detects the amino acids in the sweat is an easy and accurate method [16].

If the diagnostic studies are inconclusive or confusing, EMG and neurophysiologic studies can help establish the diagnosis and identify the nerve branches that have been injured. EMG examination attempts to differentiate between neuropraxia, axonotmesis, or neurotmesis and is outlined below.

## Electrodiagnostics

The diagnosis and prognosis of nerve injuries usually is established with electrodiagnostics. These studies are based on the principle that electrophysiologic stimulation of any nerve elicits a distal response. The site of stimulation and the resultant distal response can determine whether the injured nerve is capable of conducting a response [17]. Electrophysiologically, nerve injuries are classified as being caused by axonal loss, demyelination, or both.

When motor conduction studies are performed, the recording electrodes are placed over the muscle to be studied and a mechanical response is obtained [18]. Needle electrode examination records the electrical activity of a muscle at rest and during voluntary contraction. The patterns of electrodiagnostic abnormalities can be divided into failure of conduction, demyelinating conduction block, and conduction slowing.

In the assessment of upper extremity injuries or fractures with functional nerve loss, electrophysiologic studies are a valuable tool, especially for lesions observed to be in continuity at the time of initial assessment or when the continuity of the lesion is unknown or unobserved. The timing of the study is critical for accurate assessment of the nerve injury. Recommendations for the timing of studies include obtaining a baseline at 10 days after injury and repeating the study at 3 to 4 weeks postinjury. This protocol gives an accurate representation of the classification of the nerve injury and prognosis for recovery and represents an integral part of future treatment plans.

## Nerve injuries associated with specific fractures

Nerve injuries are associated with specific fractures of the upper extremity. These injuries can occur during the primary trauma or fracture, during the attempted reduction of the fracture, or during the surgical management of the fracture. Knowing the association of certain nerve injuries with specific fracture patterns is helpful when assessing fractures in the acute setting. Certain fractures should arouse suspicion for the possibility of nerve deficit and force the physician to perform a detailed neurovascular examination in the associated nerve distribution.

*Humerus fractures*

Nerve injuries associated with proximal humerus fractures are rare in children. Injury to the brachial plexus can result from fracture–dislocations of the proximal humerus [19]. The most common injury is to the axillary nerve after surgical neck fractures of the humerus and is related to the close proximity of this nerve to the surgical neck of the humerus [20]. The nerve commonly is spared, however, because the typical fracture pattern involves anterior and lateral angulation.

Unlike proximal humerus fractures, humeral shaft fractures have classically been associated with nerve injuries, specifically radial nerve palsies. The radial nerve lies in the spiral groove on the posterior aspect of the midshaft of the humerus and becomes fixed as it pierces the lateral intramuscular septum to enter the anterior compartment (Fig. 1). It is therefore susceptible to injury during midshaft and distal one-third fractures of the humerus when traction and angular deformities compress the nerve. The incidence of radial nerve palsies has been reported to be as high as

18% in adults, but in 90% of these injuries, nerve function returns by 4 months [21–23]. The incidence of radial nerve palsies in children has not been determined but would be assumed to be similar to the incidence in adults, given that the fracture does not involve the physis and is therefore similar in both populations. Because most radial nerve palsies are secondary to stretch or contusion, acute nerve exploration is indicated only when (1) the palsy is associated with open humeral fractures, (2) the palsy is associated with fractures requiring open reduction and internal fixation, or (3) the palsy occurs following an attempted reduction of the humerus shaft fracture [24]. Classically the occurrence of the nerve injury during an attempt at reduction of a distal third spiral oblique humerus fracture has been termed a Holstein-Lewis injury. Although there has been significant controversy surrounding whether to explore radial nerve palsies associated with humerus fracture, the current consensus is to limit exploration to the three criteria listed. This is because, although radial nerve exploration following humeral shaft fractures has shown a 12% laceration rate, similar outcomes have been reported with primary and delayed repair [25–27].

Fractures around the elbow are extremely common in children and are associated with various nerve injuries [28]. Of all fracture patterns, supracondylar humerus fractures are the most common elbow fracture in children, and more than 95% of all supracondylar fractures are extension-type injuries. In this fracture type, the direction of displacement of the distal fragment determines which nerve the spike of the proximal fragment is most likely to injure (Fig. 2). Radial nerve injuries therefore generally are associated with fractures in which the distal fragment is posteromedially displaced, whereas median nerve injuries are associated with fractures in which the distal fragment is posterolaterally displaced. A meta-analysis of 61 reports totaling 7,212 displaced fractures of the distal humerus (supracondylar) in children revealed that, although the radial nerve had been the most frequently involved nerve in older studies, more recent studies demonstrate that the median nerve is injured much more commonly, particularly the anterior interosseous nerve [5,29]. The median nerve sometimes can get entrapped in the fracture callus during the healing phase (Fig. 3A,B). The ulnar nerve is the least commonly injured nerve. Ulnar nerve palsies most frequently occur iatrogenically during pinning (Fig. 4) or with the flexion-type supracondylar fracture when the spike of the proximal fragment is directed posteriorly.

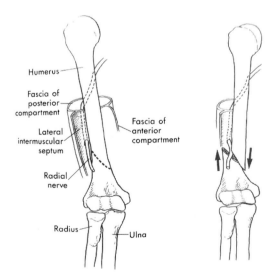

Fig. 1. Diagrammatic illustration of the anatomy of radial nerve in relation to the shaft of the humerus. The radial nerve lies in the spiral groove on the posterior aspect of the midshaft of the humerus and becomes fixed as it pierces the lateral intermuscular septum to enter the anterior compartment, thus being susceptible to injury.

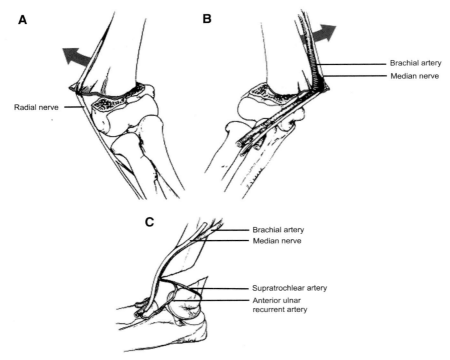

Fig. 2. Neurovascular relationship of the supracondylar fracture. (*A*) If the distal spike penetrates the brachialis muscle laterally (posteromedial fracture), the radial nerve may be tethered. (*B*) If the spike penetrates laterally (posterolateral fracture), the median nerve and brachial artery can be tethered. (*From* Kasser JR, Beaty JH. Supracondylar fractures of the distal humerus. In: Kasser JR, Beaty JH, editors. Rockwood and Wilkins' fractures in children. 5th edition. Philadelphia: Lippincott Williams and Wilkins; 2001. p. 577–624; with permission.) (*C*) The brachial artery is placed at further risk for occlusion by the ulnar-sided tether of the supratrochlear artery. (*From* Rowell PJW. Arterial occlusion in juvenile humeral supracondylar fracture. Injury 1975;6(3):254–6; with permission.)

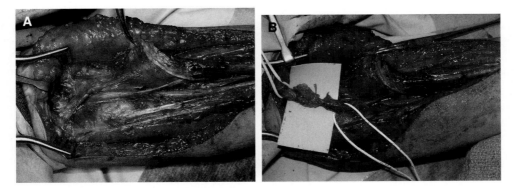

Fig. 3. This patient had a supracondylar fracture treated elsewhere by closed reduction and casting. He developed a Volkmann ischemic contracture. When the arm was explored, the median nerve was found to be entrapped in the fracture site. The nerve was freed from the bone and the injured segment was resected and repaired. (*A*) The median nerve entering the humerus. (*B*) The median nerve freed from bone.

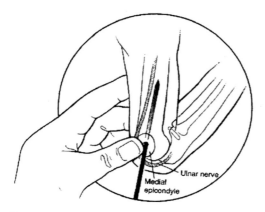

Fig. 4. Diagrammatic illustration of possible risk for damaging the ulnar nerve while pinning a supracondylar fracture. (*From* Kasser JR, Beaty JH. Supracondylar fractures of the distal humerus. In: Kasser JR, Beaty JH, editors. Rockwood and Wilkins' fractures in children. 5th edition. Philadelphia: Lippincott Williams and Wilkins; 2001. p. 577–624; with permission.)

Other fractures around the elbow are associated less commonly with nerve injuries. Acute nerve injuries after lateral condylar fractures of the humerus in children are rare, but transient radial nerve paralysis has been reported. Moreover, tardy ulnar nerve palsies can be seen secondary to lateral condyle nonunion with subsequent valgus elbow deformity. Acute ulnar nerve injury with paresthesias has been reported following medial condyle fractures of the humerus in children and is one of the relative indications for operative intervention. Furthermore, medial condyle fractures frequently are associated with elbow dislocations, and the incidence of ulnar nerve palsies in elbow dislocations has been reported to be as high as 14% [30]. Transient neuropraxia of the ulnar nerve also has been reported following metaphyseal olecranon fractures.

*Forearm fractures*

Monteggia fractures or proximal ulna fractures with associated radial head dislocations commonly are associated with various nerve palsies. The most common of these is radial nerve (10%) and posterior interosseous nerve palsy (3%–43%) [31,32]. Posterior interosseous nerve paresis is common in Monteggia fracture–dislocations associated with anterolateral dislocation of the radial head, with a high incidence of resolution in children (as compared with adults) once reduction of the radius is obtained. The ulnar nerve, tethered

by the cubital tunnel, is also at risk for injury in Monteggia fractures involving the proximal end of the ulna. The association of median nerve injuries with Monteggia fractures is low and usually anecdotal. Given that these nerve palsies are usually secondary to stretch from the radial head dislocation and not from entrapment in the ulna fracture, most will resolve with time.

Partial ulnar nerve injury and posterior interosseus nerve injury also have been reported as a direct result of radial head fracture. Most injuries to the posterior interosseous nerve occur during surgical exploration or with percutaneous pin reduction and are transient.

Forearm shaft fractures have been associated with injuries to all of the major nerves. Injuries to the median, ulnar, and posterior interosseous nerves have been reported following diaphyseal fractures of the radius–ulna, but the incidence is low because of the abundant soft-tissue protection of the nerves, and these injuries are usually transitory. Moore and colleagues, however, reported an 8.5% incidence of iatrogenic nerve injury in diaphyseal fractures that were stabilized surgically [33]. With more distal fractures, median neuropathy can occur from direct trauma secondary to the initial displacement of the distal radius fracture, traction ischemia from a persistently displaced fracture, or the development of a compartment syndrome in the carpal canal or volar

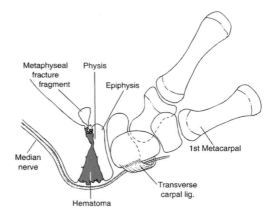

Fig. 5. Diagrammatic illustration of the anatomy outlining potential compression of the median nerve between the metaphysis of the radius and dorsally displaced physeal fracture. The tense volar transverse ligaments and fracture hematoma are also contributory. (*From* Waters PM, Kolettis GJ, Schwend R. Acute median neuropathy following physeal fractures of the distal radius. J Pediatr Orthop 1994;14(2):173–7; with permission.)

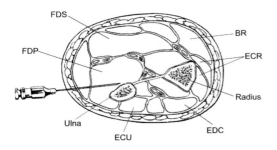

Fig. 6. Illustration of the cross-section of forearm with demonstration of different compartments. Note placement of needle to measure compartment pressures. Each compartment may be measured individually.

forearm. Median neuropathy also can occur secondary to carpal tunnel syndrome. Median and ulnar nerve injury is also common in physeal and metaphyseal fractures of the radius (Fig. 5). The mechanism of injury includes direct contusion from the displaced fragment, traction ischemia from tenting of the nerve over the proximal fragment, entrapment of the nerve in the fracture site,

rare laceration of the nerve, and the development of acute compartment syndrome. Injuries to the ulnar nerve and anterior interosseous nerve also have been described with Galeazzi fracture–dislocations and are known to have spontaneous recovery. Moore and colleagues have described an 8% incidence of injury to the radial nerve with operative exposure of the radius for internal fixation of Galeazzi fractures [33].

Distal to the elbow, the identification of various nerve injuries associated with specific fractures can be complicated by several nerve connections. The Martin-Gruber connection is a neural connection from the median or anterior interosseous nerve to the ulnar nerve in the forearm that is found in up to 23% of the population [34]. The Riche-Cannieu connection is a similar neural connection from the median nerve to the ulnar nerve that occurs in the palm. It is important to be aware of both when evaluating for nerve injuries, and their existence emphasizes the importance of doing a complete neurovascular examination in all patients in the acute fracture setting [35]. In addition, these neural

Table 2

Characteristics of acute compartment syndrome, arterial injury, nerve injury, and guidelines in an obtunded patient

| | Acute compartment syndrome | Arterial injury | Nerve injury | Guidelines in obtunded patient |
|---|---|---|---|---|
| Pain | Pain exceeding that expected from clinical situation | Less severe pain | Decreased sensation | Unreliable; pain may be obscured |
| Motor | Weakness of involved muscles | Paralysis | Decreased motor function | Unreliable; weakness may not be detectable |
| Sensory | Hypesthesia in distribution of nerves coursing through compartment | +/− sensory/motor loss | — | — |
| Vascular | Peripheral pulses frequently normal | Pulselessness +/− | Pulse intact | Unreliable in all patients |
| Stretch test | Pain on passive stretch of involved muscles | Less severe pain on passive stretch | No pain on passive stretch | Unreliable; pain may be diminished or obscured |
| Palpation | +/− tense compartment | +/− tense compartment | Compartments soft | Can be relied on to confirm other findings |
| Compartment pressure | +/− pressures elevated above normal | No pressure elevation | No pressure elevation | Pressure elevation reliable for confirming diagnosis of compartment syndrome |
| Hand position | +/− intrinsic-minus position of hand, suggesting compartment syndrome of hand | No change | No change | Intrinsic-minus position reliable for confirming diagnosis of compartment syndrome of hand |

*Adapted from* Ouellette EA. Compartment syndromes in obtunded patients. Hand Clin 1998;14(3):431–50.

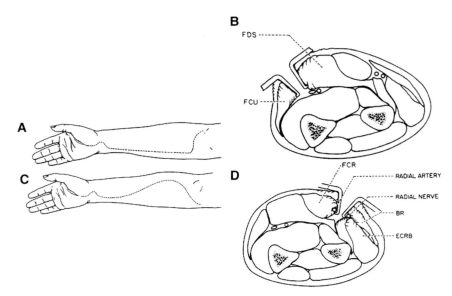

Fig. 7. Surgical approach for forearm fasciotomy. (*A*) Ulnar approach, skin incision. (*B*) Ulnar approach, intermuscular interval. (*C*) Henry approach, skin incision. (*D*) Henry approach. BR, brachioradialis; ECRB, extensor carpi radialis brevis; FCR, flexor carpi radialis; FCU, flexor carpi ulnaris; FDS, flexor digitorum superficialis. (*From* Willis RB, Roreback CH. Treatment of compartment syndrome in children. Orthop Clin North Am 1990;21(2):401–12; with permission.)

connections can explain confusing clinical scenarios after nerve injury.

### Compartment syndrome

Compartment syndrome is a symptom complex resulting from increased tissue pressure within a limited space that compromises the circulation and function of the contents of that space. Unrelieved pressure can cause progressive necrosis of muscles and nerves and eventually the skin. Necrotic muscle undergoes fibrosis and contracture. Nerve injury and damage causes further muscle dysfunction, sensory deficits, or chronic pain. The result is a dysfunctional, deformed limb known as Volkmann ischemic contracture. Crush

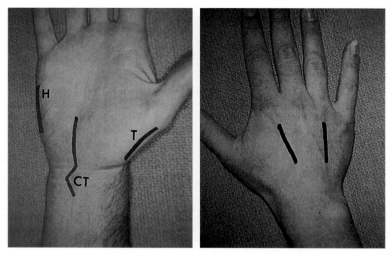

Fig. 8. Clinical picture illustrating the dorsal and volar (hypothenar, thenar, and carpal tunnel) incisions for decompression of hand compartments in compartment syndrome.

syndrome is a related term referring to a compartment syndrome that leads to systemic symptoms. In crush syndrome, muscle necrosis or rhabdomyolysis causes myoglobinemia, hyperkalemia, and acidosis that can result in renal failure, cardiac arrhythmia, shock, and even death.

Although compartment syndrome is most common in the forearm in the upper extremity, hand and upper arm compartment syndromes also have been reported. Traumatic causes (including crush injuries, prolonged external compression, fractures, and bleeding) remain the foremost etiology of compartment syndrome.

Anatomically the forearm can be divided into four identifiable interconnected compartments. These include the superficial volar compartment, the deep volar compartment, the dorsal compartment, and the compartment containing the mobile wad of Henry (brachioradialis and extensor carpi radialis longus and brevis) (Fig. 6).

The tolerance of tissue to prolonged ischemia varies according to the type of tissue. Rorabeck and Clarke have demonstrated that the duration of increased pressure is significant in the return of neurologic function. Pressures from 40 to 80 mm Hg sustained for 4 hours caused no permanent nerve dysfunction, but when applied for 12 hours or more, permanent neurologic changes occurred [36].

The early diagnosis of impending ischemia is essential. Pain is the most consistent symptom, although it may not be discovered in altered sensorium and comatose patients. Guidelines for differentiating the clinical presentation of acute compartment syndrome, arterial injury, and nerve injury in the upper extremity together with reliability features in obtunded patients are presented in Table 2 [37]. Other findings include a feeling of increased tension within the muscle compartments, increased pain with passive stretch, decreased sensibility, abnormal two-point discrimination, decreased vibration perception, and feeble or absent pulsations, although absence of these may not rule out a compartment syndrome. Diagnosis usually is confirmed by objective demonstration of increased compartment pressure (Fig. 6) and fasciotomy usually is recommended at pressures greater than 30 mm Hg or when the tissue pressures reach 30 to 10 mm Hg below the diastolic blood pressure. As a general rule, when in doubt the compartment should be released.

Common skin incisions used for compartment release in the forearm and hand are presented in Figs. 7 and 8.

### Nerve repair

Nerve repair in partial nerve injuries is directed mainly at restoring continuity of the nerve with all of its elements. Technique or method of repair is based on the location of the injury and the type and size of the nerve [38,39]. Surgical repair can be epineural, group fascicular, or fascicular (Figs. 9 and 10). Principles of nerve repair are outlined in Box 1.

### Nerve grafting

Nerve grafting in partial nerve injuries is indicated in an acute injury when there is a partial nerve defect (Fig. 11) that cannot be repaired without tension [40,41]. The procedure of nerve grafting for partial nerve injury is illustrated in Fig. 11. The main advantage of the grafting

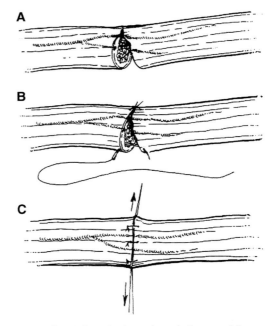

Fig. 9. Illustration of epineural repair for a partial nerve injury. The proximal and distal ends of the epineurium are approximated and continuity is restored with two or three stitches. Vessels on the epineural surface of the nerve are of great importance not only for nutrition of the nerve but also for successful orientation and must be preserved during dissection. (*A*) The nerve has been partially lacerated. (*B*) Vessels are an important guide for correct orientation. (*C*) Completed repair with injured epineural vessels correctly approximated. (*From* Varitimidis SE, Sotereanos DG. Partial nerve injuries in the upper extremity. Hand Clin 2000;16(1):141–9; with permission.)

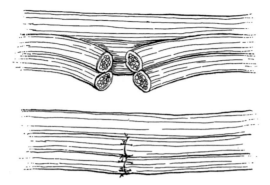

Fig. 10. Fascicular group repair. The lacerated groups are dissected and exposed proximally and distally. Each fascicular group then is repaired individually. (*From* Varitimidis SE, Sotereanos DG. Partial nerve injuries in the upper extremity. Hand Clin 2000;16(1): 141–9; with permission.)

technique is that repair is done without tension, and vascularity of the nerve is not compromised, because there is no need to mobilize the nerve to gain length. The injured segments are not stretched to reach each other, and longitudinal

---

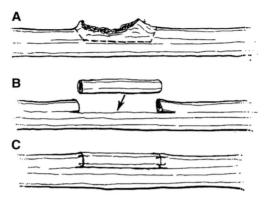

Fig. 11. Nerve grafting for partial nerve injury. (*A*) The damaged part of the nerve is removed. (*B*) A nerve graft with appropriate length compared with the defect is used to restore continuity without tension. (*C*) Repair is completed with stitches proximally and distally. (*From* Varitimidis SE, Sotereanos DG. Partial nerve injuries in the upper extremity. Hand Clin 2000;16(1):141–9; with permission.)

vasculature remains intact. Disadvantages include longer distance that the regenerating axons must travel and donor site morbidity, including the need for axons to pass two neurorrhaphy sites.

### Nerve wrapping with a vein graft

This procedure typically is performed in cases in which scar forms at the site of injury and compresses the intact fascicles. The degenerated segment is excised to expose a healthy portion of nerve. The vein is harvested, opened longitudinally, and wrapped around the nerve with its intima on the epineural surface of the nerve (Fig. 12) [41]. Injured and uninjured fascicles are wrapped. It is believed that the vein prevents excessive scar formation at the scar site. Some proponents of the technique believe that the regenerating neural axons find their way across the vein conduit because of the phenomenon of neurotropism. Vein grafts also can be used as nerve conduits in pure sensory nerve defects less than 2 cm (eg, digital nerve). Synthetic conduits are also now available.

### Summary

In every child who has a fracture, neurologic examination is essential at initial assessment so that early diagnosis of nerve injury can be made. Electrodiagnostic studies may be helpful in diagnosis when the examination is equivocal and in follow-up to look for signs of recovery. In a patient

---

**Box 1. Important principles of nerve repair**

Preparation of the nerve stump and approximation of the stumps with no tension are essential, because blood supply to the nerve, especially intraneural, may be compromised.

It is important to consider normal excursion of the nerve when the extremity is moving.

Lacerated fascicles must be dissected proximally and distally until adequate exposure is obtained for repair.

Epineural vessels must be preserved, because they serve as an important guide for fascicular orientation during repair.

Direct or primary repair of the defect is performed if the distance between nerve ends is up to approximately 2 cm and repair of the defect is performed with nerve grafts if the defect is greater than 4 cm. For defects between 2 and 4 cm, direct repair or grafting may be chosen on a case-by-case basis.

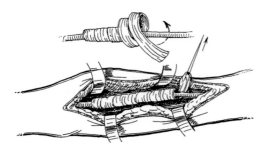

Fig. 12. Vein wrapping for a partial nerve injury. The vein is harvested, opened longitudinally, and wrapped around the nerve with its intima on the epineural surface of the nerve (*From* Varitimidis SE, Sotereanos DG. Partial nerve injuries in the upper extremity. Hand Clin 2000;16(1):141–9; with permission.)

who has neurologic deficits associated with a fracture, nerve exploration should be considered for open fractures, fractures that require open reduction, and palsies that develop after fracture reduction. For closed fractures associated with nerve palsy at the time of initial injury, observation and serial examination after reduction is recommended. If there is no return of nerve function on examination or electrodiagnostic testing by 4 months, operative exploration is indicated.

## Acknowledgments

The authors would like to thank Rebecca Gaugler, BA, Research Coordinator, Division of Orthopedic Surgery, The Children's Hospital of Philadelphia, for her assistance with this article.

## References

[1] Omer GE. Injuries to nerves of the upper extremity. J Bone Joint Surg [Am] 1974;56(8):1615–24.

[2] Hanlon CR, Estes WL. Fractures in childhood, a statistical analysis. Am J Surg 1954;87(3):312–23.

[3] Mehlman C, Crawford A, McMillion TL, et al. Operative treatment of supracondylar fractures of the humerus in children: the Cincinnati experience. Acta Orthop Belg 1996;62(Suppl 1):41–50.

[4] Sairyo K, Henmi T, Kanematsu Y, et al. Radial nerve palsy associated with slightly angulated pediatric supracondylar humerus fracture. J Orthop Trauma 1997;11(3):227–9.

[5] Kasser JR, Beaty JH. Supracondylar fractures of the distal humerus. In: Kasser JR, Beaty JH, editors. Rockwood and Wilkins' fractures in children. 5th edition. Philadelphia: Lippincott Williams and Wilkins; 2001. p. 577–624.

[6] Hill C, Riaz M, Mozzam A, et al. A regional audit of hand and wrist injuries. A study of 4873 injuries. J Hand Surg [Br] 1998;23(2):196–200.

[7] Pollock FH, Drake D, Bovill EG, et al. Treatment of radial neuropathy associated with fractures of the humerus. J Bone Joint Surg [Am] 1981;63(2):239–43.

[8] Noble J, Munro CA, Prasad VS, et al. Analysis of upper and lower extremity peripheral nerve injuries in a population of patients with multiple injuries. J Trauma 1998;45(1):116–22.

[9] Seddon HJ. Three types of nerve injury. Brain 1943; 66(4):238–83.

[10] Sunderland S. A classification of peripheral nerve injuries producing loss of function. Brain 1951;74(4): 491–516.

[11] Mackinnon SE. Peripheral nerve injuries. In: Light TR, editor. Hand surgery update 2. 1st edition. Illinois: American Society for Surgery of the Hand; 1999. p. 199–210.

[12] Flores AJ, Lavernia CJ, Owens PW. Anatomy and physiology of peripheral nerve injury and repair. Am J Orthop 2000;29(3):167–73.

[13] Seddon HJ, Holmes W. Ischemic damage in the peripheral stump of a divided nerve. Br J Surg 1945; 32:389.

[14] Sunderland S, Ray LJ. Denervation changes in mammalian striated muscle. J Neurol Neurosurg Psychiatr 1950;13(3):159–77.

[15] Woodhall B, Beebe GW. Peripheral nerve regeneration: a follow-up study of 3,156 World War II injuries. Washington, DC: US Government Printing Office; 1956.

[16] Aschan W, Moberg E. The ninhydrin finger printing test used to map out partial lesions to hand nerves. Acta Chir Scand 1962;123:365–70.

[17] Goldner JL, Nashold BS, Hendrix PC. Peripheral nerve electrical stimulation. Clin Orthop Relat Res 1982;163:33–41.

[18] Terzis JK, Dykes RW, Hakstian RW. Electrophysiological recordings in peripheral nerve surgery: a review. J Hand Surg [Am] 1976;1(1):52–66.

[19] Drew SJ, Giddins GE, Birch R. A slowly evolving brachial plexus injury following a proximal humeral fracture in a child. J Hand Surg [Br] 1995;20(1):24–5.

[20] Artico M, Salvati M, D'Andrea V, et al. Isolated lesion of the axillary nerve: surgical treatment and outcome in 12 cases. Neurosurgery 1991;29(5): 697–700.

[21] Pollock FH, Drake D, Bovill EG, et al. Treatment of radial neuropathy associated with fractures of the humerus. J Bone Joint Surg [Am] 1981;63(2):239–43.

[22] Garcia A Jr, Maeck BH. Radial nerve injuries in fractures of the shaft of the humerus. Am J Surg 1960;99:625–7.

[23] Mast JW, Spiegel PG, Harvey JP, et al. Fractures of the humeral shaft. Clin Orthop 1975;12:254–62.

[24] Ring D, Chin K, Jupiter J. Radial nerve palsy associated with high-energy humeral shaft fractures. J Hand Surg [Am] 2004;29(1):144–7.

[25] Shah JJ, Bhatti NA. Radial nerve paralysis associated with fractures of the humerus. Clin Orthop 1983;172:171–6.

[26] Packer JW, Foster RR, Garcia A, et al. The humeral fracture with radial nerve palsy: is exploration warranted? Clin Orthop 1972;88:34–8.

[27] Bostman O, Bakalim G, Vainionpaa S, et al. Radial palsy in shaft fracture of the humerus. Acta Orthop Scand 1986;57:316–9.

[28] Dormans JP, Squillante R, Sharf H. Acute neurovascular complications with supracondylar humerus fractures in children. J Hand Surg 1995;20(1): 1–4.

[29] Cramer KE, Green NE, Devito DP. Incidence of anterior interosseous nerve palsy in supracondylar humerus fractures in children. J Pediatr Orthop 1993;13(4):502–5.

[30] Linscheid RL, Wheeler DK. Elbow dislocations. JAMA 1965;194(11):1171–6.

[31] Bruce HE, Harvey JP, Wilson JC. Monteggia fractures. J Bone Joint Surg [Am] 1974;56(8): 1563–76.

[32] Jessing P. Monteggia lesions and their complicating nerve damage. Acta Orthop Scand 1975;46(4): 601–9.

[33] Moore TM, Klein JP, Patzakis MJ, et al. Results of compression-plating of closed Galeazzi fractures. J Bone Joint Surg [Am] 1985;67(7):1015–21.

[34] Rodriquez-Niedenfuhr M, Vazquez T, Parkin I, et al. Martin-Gruber anastomosis revisited. Clin Anat 2002;15(2):129–34.

[35] Amoiridis G. Median–ulnar nerve communications and anomalous innervation of the intrinsic hand muscles: an electrophysiological study. Musc Nerve 1992;15(5):576–9.

[36] Rorabeck CH, Clarke KM. The pathophysiology of the anterior tibial compartment syndrome: an experimental investigation. J Trauma 1978;18(5):299–304.

[37] Ouellette EA. Compartment syndromes in obtunded patients. Hand Clin 1998;14(3):431–50.

[38] Millesi H. Microsurgery of peripheral nerves. Hand 1973;5(2):157–60.

[39] Sunderland S. The anatomic foundation of peripheral nerve repair techniques. Orthop Clin North Am 1981;12(2):245–66.

[40] Millesi H. Interfascicular grafts for repair of peripheral nerves of the upper extremity. Orthop Clin North Am 1977;8(2):387–404.

[41] Varitimidis SE, Sotereanos DG. Partial nerve injuries in the upper extremity. Hand Clin 2000;16(1):141–9.

# Management of Established Volkmann's Contracture of the Forearm in Children

Milan Stevanovic, MD[a],*, Frances Sharpe, MD[b]

[a]Department of Orthopedics, University of Southern California Keck School of Medicine,
Los Angeles County Medical Center, 2025 Zonal Avenue, GNH Room 3900, Los Angeles, CA 90033, USA
[b]Southern California Permanente Medical Group, 9985 Sierra Avenue, Fontana, CA 92335, USA

Acute compartment syndrome and the subsequent development of Volkmann's ischemic contracture can be one of the most devastating complications of pediatric trauma. Prompt recognition and treatment of an acute compartment syndrome reduces the overall morbidity associated with this condition. However, prolonged ischemia can result in irreversible changes in the muscles, nerves, and vascular endothelium, leading to permanent disability of the hand and wrist. This end result of ischemia is what is known as *Volkmann's ischemic contracture* (Fig. 1).

## History

Richard von Volkmann (Fig. 2), in 1881, was one of the first to describe ischemic muscle paralysis and contracture [1]. Before this, a few case reports of hand and wrist deformity following injury had been described; however, paralysis and contracture were attributed to neurologic injury [2]. Volkmann was probably the first to thoroughly describe this entity and attribute the cause to muscle ischemia. He described a progressive posttraumatic muscle contracture that did not respond to splinting, and attributed the contracture to ischemia and subsequent muscle necrosis. Hildebrand, in 1890, was the first to use the term *Volkmann's contracture* [2].

Subsequent animal investigations and a thorough clinical description by Leser in 1884 brought

further attention to this condition, its presentation, and etiology. He considered the pathologic findings in the muscle to be a result of oxygen deprivation to the muscle, but did not discuss the etiology of the oxygen deprivation.

Several early investigators pursued the concept of a vascular disturbance, such as venous stasis, leading to muscle ischemia. The concept of increasing internal pressure within the forearm evolved [2–5]. This concept led Bardenheuer [4] to the idea of releasing the internal pressure through a forearm fasciotomy to treat an *impending* Volkmann's contracture. In 1926, Jepson developed an animal model that reproduced the findings of Volkmann's contracture. He used this model to show that muscle damage could be prevented by surgical decompression of pressure in the muscle compartment, although he described this as an opening of the wound with an evacuation of blood and serum [2]. By 1928, the core opinion on the etiology of contracture was that of increased pressure within the muscle compartment. The contracture was caused by pressure applied from without (ie, the tight bandaging described by Volkmann), from within, or from a combination of both [6].

The notion that arterial injury alone was the cause of ischemia gradually replaced the concept of pressure ischemia, likely because of the problems associated with arterial injuries during World War I [7,8]. This concept was supported most strongly by Griffiths, who purported that Volkmann's ischemic contracture was caused solely by arterial injury with reflex spasm of the collateral vessels. He asserted that Volkmann's initial concept of tight external bandaging was at most

* Corresponding author.
*E-mail address:* stevanov@hsc.usc.edu
(M. Stevanovic).

*hand.theclinics.com*

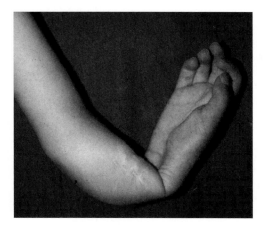

Fig. 1. Late sequelae of severe type Volkmann's ische-mic contracture.

a contributory factor [8]. This concept persisted for the next 25 years. The focus on addressing the arterial injury and spasm (and if no injury were present, performing arterial sympathectomy) supplanted almost completely the concept of pres-sure ischemia, and routine use of fasciotomies to treat impending Volkmann's contractures was abandoned. While Griffiths was in part responsible

for this setback in treatment, he should be credited for describing the early clinical signs of an impend-ing Volkmann's contracture.

Holden should be recognized for returning to the concept of addressing the intrinsic pressure within the muscle compartments. He distin-guished two patterns of injury leading to the development of Volkmann's contracture. The Type I injury results from an arterial insult proximal to the site of ischemia. The Type II injury results from a direct insult in the distal segment, resulting in localized increase in pres-sure. While the causes are different, the pattern of distal injury is constant. He emphasized the importance of not only addressing the arterial injury in the Type I pattern but also, in both Type I and Type II, addressing the elevated intrinsic pressure in the distal segment [9,10].

As the pathogenesis of ischemic contracture was better understood, treatment of impending Volkmann's ischemic contracture (acute compart-ment syndrome) became more refined. Eichler and Lipscomb [11] outlined the early technique of fas-ciotomy. Significant advances in the methods of diagnosis and monitoring of compartment pres-sures were introduced by Whitesides, Hargens, Mubarak, and Matsen [12–15]. Refinements in surgical technique were described further by Ea-ton and Green, Whitesides, Gelberman, and others [15–17]. The recognition and treatment of acute compartment syndrome have greatly dimin-ished the incidence and severity of Volkmann's is-chemic contracture.

**Pathophysiology**

Volkmann's ischemic contracture is the end result of prolonged ischemia of the muscles and nerves in an extremity. Most commonly, this is caused by untreated or prolonged ischemia from an acute compartment syndrome. High tissue fluid pressures within a muscle compartment reduce capillary perfusion below a level necessary for tissue survival. Sustained ischemia can result in irreversible changes to the muscle, which un-dergoes necrosis. The necrotic muscle is replaced with fibrotic tissue, clinically presenting as contracture.

Experimental studies have produced irrevers-ible muscle necrosis after 4 hours of ischemia [12,18]. In the forearm, the pattern of necrosis in-volves an elliptically shaped area in the middle third of the forearm [19]. The necrotic muscle is

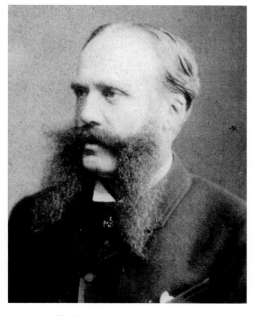

Fig. 2. Richard von Volkmann.

replaced by fibroblasts, which cause adhesions to the surrounding tissue and contract in both longitudinal and horizontal planes. The maturation of the fibrotic tissue occurs over 6 months to a year, allowing the severity of the clinical contracture to progress over this time. Permanent nerve injury can occur from the initial insult. More nerve impairment occurs as the necrotic muscle becomes more fibrotic and compresses the nerve. Nerve function is impaired further by the inability of the nerve to glide through a fibrotic tissue bed. Nerve circulation is also diminished by the dense fibrotic tissue. On surgical exploration, the nerve can be markedly constricted and atrophic, with the appearance of a thin line of tissue. Dissection of the nerve through this dense scar tissue and extensive neurolysis may result in further neurologic injury.

## Clinical presentation

The clinical presentation of acute compartment syndrome differs from that of the established Volkmann's contracture. Diagnosis of acute compartment syndrome remains principally a clinical diagnosis. Certain types of injuries should raise the index of suspicion for the development of compartment syndrome. In children, the most frequent injury associated with compartment syndrome is the displaced supracondylar fracture of the humerus [14,20,21]. With the increased use of closed reduction and pinning for supracondylar humerus fractures, the incidence of compartment syndrome associated with this injury has decreased [22]. Diaphyseal forearm fractures are also a frequently associated injury, with 15% to 22% of ischemic contractures occurring as a complication of forearm fracture [14,22–24]. In the authors' experience, those fractures with combined fracture of the distal radius are at a much higher risk of developing an acute compartment syndrome. This was found as well by Blakemore and colleagues [25], who cited a 33% incidence of acute compartment syndrome in cases with displaced fractures of the distal humerus and an associated displaced forearm fracture. Also, cast immobilization with the elbow at 90 degrees or more of flexion has been a common associated finding. The hallmark of diagnosis is a swollen, tense, and tender compartment that does not improve with elevation.

Several authors have described additional clinical findings associated with the diagnosis of compartment syndrome. Over time these have been refined to the "5 p's" of diagnosis:

- *Pain.* Pain is out of proportion to the injury, often causing a patient to have a progressively increasing narcotic requirement. Even with increasing pain medications, the pain is not relieved.
- *Pain with passive motion.* Passive stretching of the fingers or wrist causes pain in the ischemic compartment.
- *Pallor.* This has been seen in some cases. Usually this is associated with a proximal vascular compromise affecting the brachial artery. This may be tenting of the artery across the fracture site, arterial spasm due to adjacent trauma, or arterial thrombosis secondary to intimal injury.
- *Pulselessness.* This can be associated with pallor. Pulselessness is a rare finding and usually occurs late in the diagnosis.
- *Paresthesia and paralysis.* These conditions are variably present. Jepson [2] stated that "within a few hours, the patient complains that the fingers are numb. The patient is usually more concerned than the surgeon." Although numbness and paresthesias have been described as the first clinical finding [26,27], the authors' experience is that these may or may not be present, and when present occur late. Further, eliciting this information from a child may be difficult and unreliable. Sensory findings of dysthesia, hypesthesia, or anesthesia caused by a compartment syndrome are distal to the affected compartment. Sensory findings usually precede motor findings.

In obtunded patients or patients who suffer neurologic injury, clinical findings may be difficult to elicit. Careful and repeated clinical examination and monitoring of compartment pressures using any of several methods can aid in diagnosis. The authors have a low threshold for surgical decompression of a suspected compartment syndrome. In children, it is often better to measure compartment pressures in the operating room, as it is far less traumatizing to the child and to the parents. If a compartment syndrome is present, immediate treatment with fasciotomy should be performed. The potential complications from a fasciotomy that might not have been necessary are far less than the complications from an untreated compartment syndrome.

A unique category of presentation is that of the neonatal Volkmann's contracture. Perhaps it should be better named neonatal compartment syndrome. This condition is quite rare, principally described in case reports [28–33]. In a recent retrospective review, Ragland and coauthors [34] identified 24 patients over a 20-year period who had clinical evidence of forearm ischemia at the time of birth. These neonates had been recognized subsequently to have had an acute or subacute compartment syndrome with impending Volkmann's ischemia. Often this was not identified initially and most children developed later contracture, deformity, and extremity dysfunction. These investigators highlight the importance of early recognition and treatment, and suggest that neonatal Volkmann's ischemia be renamed as neonatal compartment syndrome, emphasizing the importance of emergent intervention. An important diagnostic finding was that of sentinel forearm skin lesion, which should alert the physician to the possibility of an underlying ischemia, in which instance immediate surgical treatment is necessary.

Established Volkmann's contracture has a much different presentation. It has a broad clinical spectrum, based on the extent of muscle necrosis and nerve injury that has occurred. The deformity results from the ischemic event and subsequent muscle fibrosis and nerve dysfunction, either from the initial insult or secondary to the subsequent scarring and vascular compromise to the nerve. The deformity therefore occurs over a period of weeks to months. Untreated deformity in a child will progress until skeletal maturity.

The most vulnerable muscle group is the deep flexor compartment of the forearm, which includes the flexor digitorum profundus (FDP) muscle and the flexor pollicis longus (FPL). In the mildest form of ischemic contracture, it is these muscles that are affected, and often only a portion of these muscles. Typically, the ring and long fingers are the most commonly affected profundus muscles. Next most common is the FPL, followed by the index and small fingers [35–37]. The flexor digitorum superficialis, pronator teres, and wrist flexors are involved with more severe or prolonged ischemia. In the most severe cases, ischemia and subsequent necrosis of the extensor compartment can occur as well. As the area of necrosis expands, there is greater involvement of the nerves. The median nerve is more susceptible to ischemia and subsequent fibrosis than the ulnar nerve. In severe cases, the posture of the wrist is in flexion, sometimes with associated forearm pronation. The position of the fingers is variable, ranging from a simple claw deformity with

flexion of the metacarpophalangeal and interphalangeal joints to an intrinsic plus or intrinsic minus posture, depending on the involvement of the ulnar nerve or the involvement of the hand intrinsic muscles. The intrinsic minus deformity is seen more commonly than the intrinsic plus deformity because of the greater strength of the extrinsic flexor and extensor muscles. Flexion of the wrist usually allows active and passive extension of the fingers. However, chronic muscle imbalance and failure to maintain passive range of motion lead to stiff and contracted joints [35,38].

It is important to distinguish a true Volkmann's contracture from a pseudo-Volkmann's contracture. Pseudo-Volkmann's is caused most commonly by entrapment or tethering of the FDP or the FPL to the fractures of the radius or ulna. Other causes include adhesions around internal fixation, tendon rupture, crush injury, and scarring secondary to infection [39]. Clinically, this can be very difficult to distinguish from a true Volkmann's contracture, especially from a mild Volkmann's ischemia [39,40]. At surgical exploration, the muscles will appear normal, but adherent to the bone. A myotenolysis or tenolysis alone will usually allow correction. Because muscle entrapment at the fracture site is one of the more frequent causes of pseudo-Volkmann's, it is important to check passive range of motion of the digits following reduction. Extension is affected most commonly due to entrapment of the deep flexors. This can be corrected easily with open reduction of the fracture.

## Classification

Several classification systems have been described, with considerable overlap. Most are based on the clinical severity of the presentation and are used to help direct the appropriate treatment for the identified disability. Most investigators recognize the tremendous variability of the clinical presentations and the subsequent limitations of the classification systems [36–38,41,42].

Seddon [41] was the first to introduce the concept of the ellipsoid infarct involving the muscles of the proximal forearm (Fig. 3). He further described a spectrum of contracture from mild to severe. The mild type responds to splinting with little to no residual sequelae, with the possible recurrence of contracture as a young child grows to maturity. The most severe type was described as

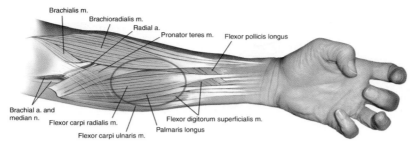

Fig. 3. Ellipsoid zone of injury as described by Seddon.

a limb that "apart from its envelope is gangrenous and whose treatment is futile." Between these two extremes, he described three separate patterns of presentation:

- Diffuse but moderate ischemia. The main feature in this presentation is contracture. Nerve involvement is limited and resolves spontaneously. Most function returns spontaneously, and at the end of a few months there is left only residual contracture to correct.
- Intense but localized muscle damage. This occurs rarely, but with a distinct presentation in which the primary involvement is that of the deep flexors of the forearm, specifically FDP and FPL. Minimal involvement of the median nerve adjacent to the zone of infarction can also be present.
- Widespread necrosis or fibrosis. In this presentation there is near total destruction of all the muscles of the forearm. The median and ulnar nerve function is compromised, and there may be extension of the infarct into the dorsal compartment.

As noted by Zancolli [38], there is significant variability in the involvement of the hand. His classification system was based entirely on the involvement of the intrinsic muscles. Type I cases have no intrinsic involvement (simple claw deformity). In Type II deformity, the intrinsic muscles are paralyzed, resulting in an intrinsic minus claw hand and opponens paralysis. Type III deformity is defined by intrinsic muscle contracture with the clinical appearance of an intrinsic plus hand and intrinsic plus thumb. In the Type IV combined group, there is a mixed presentation of intrinsic involvement. At times there may be some fingers with an intrinsic minus posture (usually the 4th and 5th fingers), with an intrinsic plus posture affecting the adjacent fingers (usually the index and middle). The variability in presentation

depends on the ischemic insult and potential recovery to the median and ulnar nerves, and there is no uniform pattern to predict whether the thenar or hypothenar muscles will be spared or the extent of the intrinsic paresis or paralysis.

Perhaps the most commonly used classification system is that of Tsuge [36]. He classified established Volkmann's contracture into *mild*, *moderate*, and *severe* types, according to the extent of the muscle involvement. This is the authors' preferred method of classification.

The mild type, also described as the localized type, involves the muscles of the deep flexor compartment of the forearm, usually involving only the FDP of the ring or middle fingers (Fig. 4A). It can involve all the FDP and the FPL as well. Nerve involvement is absent or mild, typically consisting of sensory changes which resolve spontaneously. With wrist flexion, the fingers can be fully extended. Most of the mild type result from direct trauma, either from crush injury or forearm fractures, and are typically seen in young adults.

In the moderate type, the muscle degeneration includes all or nearly all of the FDP and FPL, with partial degeneration of the flexor superficialis muscles (Fig. 4B). Neurologic impairment is always present. Sensory impairment is generally more severe in the median than in the ulnar nerve, and the hand demonstrates an intrinsic minus posture. Moderate-type injury is most commonly the result of supracondylar humerus fractures in children between ages 5 and 10.

The severe type involves degeneration of all the flexor muscles of the fingers and the wrist. There is central muscle necrosis, and varying involvement of the extensor compartment (Fig. 4C). Neurological deficits are severe, including complete palsy of all the intrinsic muscles of the hand. Tsuge categorized those cases that may have had moderate involvement initially but, because of fixed joint

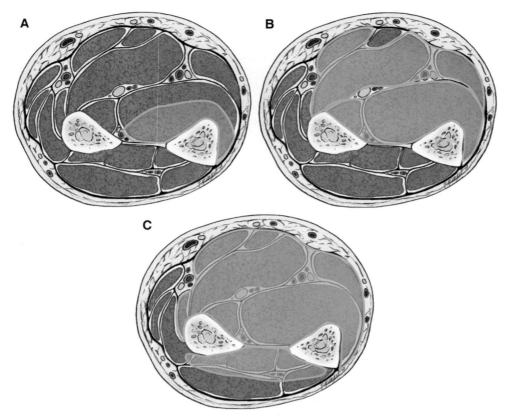

Fig. 4. Cross-section of mid-forearm with lighter shaded area demonstrating area of infarction. (*A*) Mild type, with infarction of flexor digitorum profundus and flexor pollicis longus. (*B*) Moderate (classic) type, with infarction of flexor digitorum superficials and profundus, flexor pollicis longus, and wrist flexors and pronator. (*C*) Severe type, with flexor and extensor compartment involvement.

contractures, scarred soft tissue envelope, or failed surgeries, were categorized as severe. As with moderate cases, severe cases are most commonly the result of supracondylar humerus fractures in children.

Within each classification type, there is a broad range of clinical presentation. This heterogeneity of presentation makes it difficult to apply a specific treatment based solely on classification systems, and makes it nearly impossible to provide meaningful outcome and comparison studies.

### Treatment

Treatment of an impending Volkmann's ischemic contracture is quite different from treating an established contracture. Acute compartment syndrome should be treated with emergent fasciotomy as soon as the condition is identified.

Controversy persists regarding treatment in the late acute phase, when an elevated compartment pressure has been present for more than 48 hours [37,43,44]. Some investigators recommend only a limited fasciotomy, without performing an extensive neurolysis or exploration of the nerves. The reluctance to perform extensive surgical exploration at this stage is due to concern about creating more extensive scarring and potential injury to the compromised tissues, including the nerves. Additionally, there is a concern about the increased risk of infection caused by exposing the necrotic tissue with a poor soft-tissue envelope.

The authors recommend release of the fascial compartments even in the late acute phase (2–10 days). This may improve perfusion of ischemic, but not infracted, muscle. Also, this allows the identification of early liquefactive necrosis of the muscles. When this is present, the authors think early wide excision of the nonviable muscle should be performed, and the muscle deficit reconstructed with a free functional muscle transfer. The identification of the donor vessels and donor nerves is much easier during this period, before scarring and fibrosis occurs. The authors also think this improves the soft-tissue bed and vascularity around the median and ulnar nerves, and may reduce the degree of distal neurologic deficit.

Elevation, edema control, and early static splinting should be used during the healing process. Static splinting should be continued after fracture healing. However, contracture of the fingers will often progress despite the use of these splints. Functional improvement with recovery of sensory and motor function can be seen for up to 1 year [24]. The mildest contractures can improve with splinting and a consistent program of occupational therapy. In children, these contractures may recur with skeletal growth, since the fibrotic muscle cannot adequately increase in length. Even recurrent contractures may benefit from therapy, and recurrent contractures may be prevented by the use of nighttime stretching splints used until skeletal maturity.

Once the patient has an established contracture in which soft-tissue equilibrium is present, the next phase of treatment depends on the severity of the contracture, the neurologic deficit, and the resultant functional losses.

### Nonsurgical management

Nonsurgical management should be instituted early in most cases of established Volkmann's contracture. In children, there may be more recovery of nerve and muscle function over time. The authors do not advocate immediate surgical intervention in children, with the exception noted above for severe cases when early liquefactive necrosis is present. A formal program of splinting and therapy can improve the outcome of later surgical intervention and may result in less extensive surgical corrections. Therapy should be directed toward maintenance of passive joint motion, preservation and strengthening of remaining muscle function, and correction of deformity through a program of splinting. Alternating dynamic and static splinting has been advocated. However, the authors prefer the use of static progressive splinting for fixed contractures of the wrist, fingers, and thumb web space. Mild contractures with minimal to no nerve involvement can often be treated only with

a comprehensive program of hand therapy and rehabilitation. Even for moderate to severe involvement, long-term customized splinting may be necessary to augment hand function.

### Surgical treatment

A variety of surgical procedures have been used to treat Volkmann's ischemic contracture. These have included both bone and soft-tissue management. Shortening of the radius and ulna has been used to match the bone length with the shortened fibrotic muscle [26]. Proximal row carpectomy has also been used to shorten the length of the forearm and to correct fixed flexion contractures of the wrist [45]. In general, the authors do not like shortening procedures, particularly in children, since the forearm is already relatively shortened by the initial ischemic insult to the bone and growth plates. Further, the principal contracture is usually on the flexor surface. Shortening the forearm indiscriminately lengthens the muscle resting length of both the flexor and extensor muscles, neglecting the variable involvement of the flexor compartment and the usual absence of involvement of the extensor compartment. Reconstructive bone procedures for long-standing contractures or for distal reconstruction required for neurologic injury include wrist fusion, trapeziometacarpal joint fusion, or thumb metacarpophalangeal joint fusion, which should be done after skeletal maturity. These may be considered in conjunction with some of the soft-tissue procedures listed below.

Soft-tissue procedures have included excision of the infarcted muscle, fractional or z-lengthening of the affected muscles, muscle sliding operations (flexor origin muscle slide), neurolysis, tendon transfers, and functional free muscle transfers, as well as combinations of the above procedures (see Refs. [11,19,27,36,37,43,45–52]). Excision of scarred fibrotic nerves without distal function, followed by nerve grafting, has been described to try to establish some protective sensation in the hand [53]. Fixed contractures of the joints can be addressed with soft-tissue release, including capsulectomy and collateral ligament recession or excision, depending on the joints involved.

### Preferred methods

The authors' preferred methods of treatment depend on the general classification of severity of contracture, individualized to the patient presentation.

*Mild (localized) type*

For mild contractures that have failed to respond to nonsurgical management, the authors' preferred treatment is a muscle sliding operation initially described by Page [54] and subsequently used and endorsed by several others (see Refs. [19,36,37,41,49,55,56]). Some investigators have advocated this procedure only when there is good intact distal musculature [49]. However, the authors have found this procedure effective as long as there is clinically good finger flexion evident. The authors do not combine this procedure with infarct excision; nor have we found it necessary to release the distal insertion of the pronator teres to correct pronation contracture [37,49].

The authors differ with Tsuge in our surgical incision and favor the technique initially described by Page (Fig. 5). The surgical incision begins on the ulnar distal arm and continues along the ulnar border of the forearm all the way to the wrist. The ulnar nerve is identified and mobilized. The flexor pronator mass is elevated off the medial epicondyle, taking care to preserve the medial collateral ligament and elbow joint capsule. The origins of the flexor carpi ulnaris, FDP, and flexor digitorum superficialis are carefully mobilized off the ulna and interosseous membrane, gradually heading toward the radius, with careful attention to protecting the anterior interosseous nerve and artery (Fig. 6). The anterior interosseous artery will pierce the interosseous membrane between the mid- and distal forearm, and can be injured easily in this area. A consistent branch from the ulnar artery to the posterior interosseous artery, which pierces the intermuscular septum in the proximal forearm, is also identified and spared (Fig. 7E). Working toward the radius, the origin of the FPL is progressively released. Throughout the

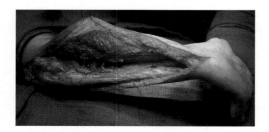

Fig. 5. Our preferred surgical approach, as originally described by Page.

procedure, the wrist and fingers are manipulated to check the degree of correction achieved and to help localize any remaining tightness within the muscle origin. Often, the dissection must be carried down to the level of the wrist before full correction is achieved. Slight undercorrection, which can be addressed by postoperative splinting and rehabilitation, may lessen the diminishment in muscle power resulting from the muscle slide. When a pronation contracture is present and not corrected by the release of the flexor-pronator origin, the authors release the pronator quadratus from the distal ulna. Even with a complete release of both pronators and dorsal distal radioulnar joint capsule, complete correction of the pronation deformity may not be possible because of fibrosis and contracture of the interosseous membrane. At the completion of the muscle slide, the ulnar nerve is transposed to an anterior subcutaneous position. The hand is splinted and subsequently casted in a position of forearm supination with wrist and finger extension. The authors continue this immobilization for a period of 6 weeks to allow the flexor pronator origin to heal adequately to its newly found origin. A limited flexor slide may be done for mild deformity, affecting only a portion of the FDP. In this case, the surgical incision is the same; however, the flexor pronator mass does not have to be released from the medial epicondyle, and the ulnar nerve does not have to be mobilized and transposed. The authors do not usually perform a neurolysis since by definition of the mild type there is little to no nerve involvement. The authors think this surgical approach limits potential scarring and vascular compromise to the remaining muscles and nerves in the flexor compartment, and the superficial veins are better preserved in the subcutaneous tissue (Fig. 7).

*Moderate type*

For moderate deformity, the authors still prefer the muscle slide operation to correct the tightness of the flexors, provided there is still adequate remaining strength in the flexors. Since neurological impairment is characteristic of the moderate injury, we combine the flexor slide with neurolysis of both the median and ulnar nerves. A separate incision to release the carpal tunnel may also be done. Depending on the functional deficits, tendon transfer can be combined with flexor slide, usually as a staged procedure. For reconstruction of thumb flexion, the authors use either brachioradialis or extensor carpi radialis longus to the FPL.

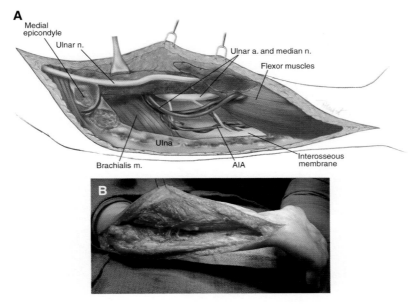

Fig. 6. (*A*) Flexor slide showing detachment of the flexor-pronator muscle origin off the medial epicondyle and supraperiosteal dissection off of the ulna. (*B*) Intraoperative photograph showing the same.

Extensor indicis proprius is used for thumb opposition. When the finger flexors are very weak or absent, a functional free-muscle transfer may produce a better functional result. When sensory impairment is severe and there has been no recovery, the nerve should be evaluated carefully at surgery. If there is a densely scarred atrophic nerve, resection of the nerve to healthy-appearing fascicles, followed by nerve graft reconstruction, may restore protective sensation to the hand.

*Severe type*

Severe type contractures are best treated with functional free-muscle transfers [43,46–48,52,57]. The donor vessel is usually either the radial, ulnar, or brachial artery. The best donor motor nerve is the anterior interosseous nerve, which should be resected back to healthy-appearing fascicles. The authors' preference for the donor muscle is the gracilis. Appropriate marking of the muscle resting length and establishment of a strong muscle origin and insertion are critical to achieving good functional results [58] (Fig. 8A–D). Zucker and colleagues [52] have described the use of separate motor fascicles of the gracilis to restore independent FDP and FPL motor function.

For severe-type contractures with extensive involvement of the extensor compartment, a double free-muscle transfer should be considered. As with the moderate type, tendon transfer, nerve graft reconstruction, and late osseous reconstructive procedures may improve final functional outcomes.

**Outcomes**

Outcomes are difficult to assess in this group of patients. Studies are limited by small numbers of patients, great variability in initial presentations, use of various surgical techniques, and difficulty in compliance with the long-term follow-up necessary to track patients through skeletal maturity. Ultee and Hovius [21] attempted to provide some information regarding outcomes. They found that all patients who had developed the contracture during childhood had a relatively shortened extremity. Substantial improvements in hand function were noted in those patients who underwent functional free-muscle transfer. Tendon lengthening alone often resulted in recurrence of contracture. Finally, in patients who had sufficient remaining muscle, procedures that combined infarct excision, tenolysis, neurolysis, and tendon transfer when necessary produced good hand function. Sundararaj and Mani [24] noted improvement in sensory function in conjunction with neurolysis. Additional procedures were done simultaneously, but little analysis of outcomes of those other procedures was given.

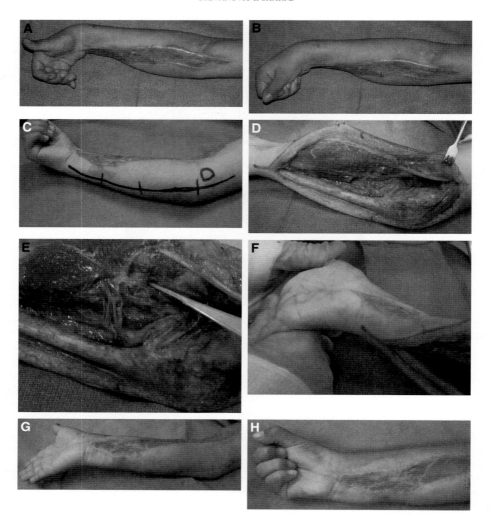

Fig. 7. A 5-year-old boy who sustained a Gartland Type III supracondylar humerus fracture with an ipsilateral distal radius fracture. He was treated with closed reduction and percutaneous pinning of the humerus and casting of the radius. Six hours later, the patient developed signs of compartment syndrome and was returned immediately to the operating room, where a fasciotomy was performed. Exploration of the brachial artery demonstrated a severely contused brachial artery with thrombosis. An interpositional vein graft was used to reconstruct the brachial artery. Despite early intervention, the patient developed a moderate-type Volkmann's ischemic contracture. After 9 months of occupational therapy and splinting, he was left with residual contracture. (A) Preoperative extension. (B) Preoperative flexion. (C) Surgical approach. (D) Intraoperative release of contracture. (E) Preserved branch from the ulnar artery traversing the interosseous membrane in the proximal forearm to anastomose with the posterior interosseous artery. (F) Intraoperative full extension of the wrist and fingers following release. (G) Postoperative extension, 6 months after surgery. (H) Postoperative flexion, 6 months after surgery.

## Summary

As with many diagnoses in medicine, the best treatment for Volkmann's ischemic contracture is prevention. Early recognition and prompt treatment of impending Volkmann's ischemia should decrease the presentation and severity of late contracture and hand dysfunction. The authors have found the flexor muscle slide the best treatment option for mild and moderate deformity. This procedure can be combined with additional reconstructive procedures to maximize

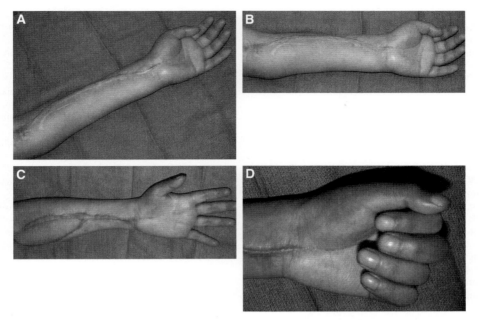

Fig. 8. A 7-year-old boy who sustained a Gartland Type III supracondylar fracture that was treated surgically two days after injury, with closed reduction and percutaneous pinning of the humerus. One day later the patient developed severe compartment syndrome. He underwent an immediate fasciotomy. He subsequently developed an infection of the open fasciotomy site. After multiple debridements to control infection, his entire flexor compartment of the forearm was eventually completely excised. Four months later, the patient underwent surgery for a functional free gracilis transfer. (*A*) Preoperative extension. (*B*) Preoperative flexion. (*C*) Nine month postoperative extension. (*D*) Nine month postoperative flexion.

functional outcome. The authors believe this procedure results in the best preservation of the muscle resting length and limits the scarring around the adjacent muscles. For severe cases, early wide excision with functional free-muscle transfer may limit the injury to the nerves, decreasing the distal problems associated with motor and sensory impairment in the hand.

## References

[1] Volkmann R. Die ischaemischen muskellaehmungen und kontrakturen. Centrabl f Chir 1881;51: 801.

[2] Jepson P. Ischaemic contracture. Experimental study. Ann Surg 1926;84(6):785–93.

[3] Murphy J. Myositis. JAMA 1914;63:1249–55.

[4] Bardenheuer L. Die entstehung und behandlung der ischaemishen muskelkontractur und gangran. Dtsch Z Chir 1911;108:44.

[5] Trice M, Colwell C. A historical review of compartment syndrome and Volkmann's ischemic contracture. Hand Clin 1998;14(3):335–41.

[6] Jones R. Volkmann's ischaemic contracture with special reference to treatment. BMJ 1928;2:639–42.

[7] Leriche R. Surgery of the sympathetic system. Indications and results. Ann Surg 1928;88:449.

[8] Griffiths D. Volkmann's ischaemic contracture. Br J Surg 1940;28:239–60.

[9] Holden C. Compartmental syndromes following trauma. Clin Orthop Relat Res 1975;113:95–102.

[10] Holden C. The pathology and prevention of Volkmann's ischaemic contracture. J Bone Joint Surg Br 1979;61B(3):296–300.

[11] Eichler G, Lipscomb P. The changing treatment of Volkmann's ischemic contractures from 1955–1965 at the Mayo Clinic. Clin Orthop Relat Res 1967; 50:215–23.

[12] Hargens A, Schmidt DA, Evans KL, et al. Quantitation of skeletal muscle necrosis in a model compartment syndrome. J Bone Joint Surg Am 1981;63A(4): 631–6.

[13] Matsen FA III, Mayo KA, Sheridan GW, et al. Continuous monitoring of intramuscular pressure and its application to clinical compartment syndromes. Bibl Anat 1977;15(1):112–5.

[14] Mubarak S, Carroll N. Volkmann's contracture in children: aetiology and prevention. J Bone Joint Surg Br 1979;61B(3):285–93.

[15] Whitesides T, Haney T, Morimoto K, et al. Tissue pressure measurement as determinant for the

need of fasciotomy. Clin Orthop Relat Res 1975; 113:43.

[16] Eaton R, Green W. Epimysiotomy and fasciotomy in the treatment of Volkmann's ischemic contracture. Orthop Clin North Am 1972;3(1):175–86.

[17] Gelberman R, Zakaib GS, Mubarak SJ, et al. Decompression of forearm compartment syndromes. Clin Orthop Relat Res 1978;134:225–9.

[18] Brooks B. Pathologic changes in muscle as a result of disturbances of circulation. Arch Surg 1922;5: 188–216.

[19] Seddon H. Volkmann's contracture: treatment by excision of the infarct. J Bone Joint Surg Br 1956; 38B(1):152–74.

[20] Eaton R, Green W. Volkmann's ischemia: a volar compartment syndrome of the forearm. Clin Orthop Relat Res 1975;113:58–64.

[21] Ultee J, Hovius S. Functional results after treatment of Volkmann's ischemic contracture: a long term followup study. Clin Orthop Relat Res 2005; 431:42–9.

[22] Kadiyala R, Waters P. Upper extremity pediatric compartment syndromes. Hand Clin 1998;14(3): 467–75.

[23] Matsen FA III, Veith R. Compartmental syndromes in children. J Pediatr Orthop 1981;1:33.

[24] Sundararaj G, Mani K. Pattern of contracture and recovery following ischaemia of the upper limb. J Hand Surg [Br] 1985;10B(2):155–61.

[25] Blakemore L, Cooperman DR, Thompson GH, et al. Compartment syndrome in ipsilateral humerus and forearm fractures in children. Clin Orthop Relat Res 2000;376:32–8.

[26] Rolands R, Lond M. A case of Volkmann's contracture treated by shortening of the radius and ulna. Lancet 1905;2:1168–71.

[27] Gulgonen A. Surgery for Volkmann's ischaemic contracture. J Bone Joint Surg Br 2001;26B(4): 283–96.

[28] Bedbrook G. Neo-natal Volkmann's syndrome. Proc R Soc Med 1953;46(5):349.

[29] Caouette-LaBerge L, Bortoluzzi P, Egerszegi EP, et al. Neonatal Volkmann's ischemic contracture of the forearm: a report of five cases. Plast Reconstr Surg 1992;90(4):621–8.

[30] Engel J, Heim M, Tsur H. Late complications of neonatal Volkmann's ischaemia. Hand 1982;14(2): 162–3.

[31] Kline S, Moore J. Neonatal compartment syndrome. J Hand Surg [Am] 1992;17A(2):256–9.

[32] Silfen R, Amir A, Sirota L, et al. Congenital Volkmann-Leser ischemic contracture of the upper limb. Ann Plast Surg 2000;45(3):313–7.

[33] Tsur H, Yaffe B, Engel Y. Impending Volkmann's contracture in a newborn. Ann Plast Surg 1980; 5(4):317–20.

[34] Ragland R III, Moukoko D, Ezaki M, et al. Forearm compartment syndrome in the newborn: report of 24 cases. J Hand Surg [Am] 2005;30(5):997–1003.

[35] Botte M, Keenan M, Gelberman R. Volkmann's ischemic contracture of the upper extremity. Hand Clin 1998;14(3):483–97.

[36] Tsuge K. Treatment of established Volkmann's contracture. J Bone Joint Surg Am 1975;57A(7): 925–9.

[37] Tsuge K. Management of established Volkmann's contracture. In: Green D, editor. Green's operative hand surgery. Philadelphia: Churchill Livingstone; 1999. p. 592–603.

[38] Zancolli E. Classification of established Volkmann's ischemic contracture and the program for its treatment. In: Zancolli E, editor. Structural and Dynamic Bases of Hand Surgery. Philadelphia: JB Lippincott; 1979.

[39] Littlefield W, Hastings H II, Strickland J. Adhesions between muscle and bone after forearm fracture mimicking mild Volkmann's ischemic contracture. J Hand Surg [Am] 1992;17A(4):691–3.

[40] Deeney V, Kaye JJ, Geary SP, et al. Pseudo-Volkmann's contracture due to tethering of flexor digitorum profundus to fractures of the ulna in children. J Pediatr Orthop 1998;18:437–40.

[41] Seddon H. Volkmann's ischaemia. BMJ 1964;1: 1587–92.

[42] Benkeddache Y, Gottesman H, Hamidani M. Proposal of a new classification for established Volkmann's contracture. Ann Chir 1985;4(2):134–42.

[43] Chuang D-C, Carver N, Wei F-C. A new strategy to prevent the sequelae of severe Volkmann's ischemia. Plast Reconstr Surg 1996;98(6):1023–31.

[44] Osborne A, Dorey L, Harvey JP Jr. Volkmann's contracture associated with prolonged external pressure on the forearm. Arch Surg 1972;104(6): 794–8.

[45] Goldner J. Volkmann's ischemic contracture. In: Flynn J, editor. Hand surgery. New York: Williams & Wilkins; 1975. p. 599–618.

[46] Chuang D-C. Functioning free-muscle transplantation for the upper extremity. Hand Clin 1997;13(2): 279–89.

[47] Ikuta Y, Kubo T, Tsuge K. Free muscle transplantation by microsurgical technique to treat severe Volkmann's contracture. Plast Reconstr Surg 1976;58(4): 407–11.

[48] Krimmer H, Hahn P, Lanz U. Free gracilis muscle transplantation for hand reconstruction. Clin Orthop Relat Res 1995;314:13–8.

[49] Lanz U, Felderhoff J. Ischaemische kontrakturen an unterarm und hand. Handchir Mikrochir Plast Chir 2000;32:6–25.

[50] Reigstad A, Hellum C. Volkmann's ischaemic contracture of the forearm. Injury 1981;12(2): 148–50.

[51] Sundararaj G, Mani K. Management of Volkmann's ischaemic contracture of the upper limb. J Bone Joint Surg Br 1985;10B(3):401–3.

[52] Zucker R, Egerszegi EP, Manktelow RT, et al. Volkmann's ischemic contracture in children: the results

of free vascularized muscle transplantation. J Micro-surg 1991;12:341–5.

[53] Hovius S, Ultee J. Volkmann's ischemic contracture. Prevention and treatment. Hand Clin 2000;16(4): 647–57.

[54] Page C. An operation for the relief of flexion-con-tracture in the forearm. J Bone Joint Surg Am 1923;3:233–4.

[55] Scaglietti O. Chirurgische behandlung der Volkmann ischaemischen paralyse. Verh Dtsch Orthop Ges 1957;45:219.

[56] Nisbet N. Volkmann's ischaemic contracture benefited by muscle slide operation: report of a case. J Bone Joint Surg Br 1952;34B(2):245–7.

[57] Liu XY, Ge BF, Win YM, et al. Free medial gastrocnemius myocutaneous flap transfer with neurovascular anastomosis to treat Volkmann's contracture of the forearm. Br J Plast Surg 1992; 45:6–8.

[58] Stevanovic M, Sharpe F. Functional free gracilis transfer for upper extremity reconstruction. Atlas Hand Clin 2002;7(1):163–80.

# Wrist Deformities After Fracture

## Ann VanHeest, MD[a,b,c,*]

[a]*Department of Orthopaedic Surgery, University of Minnesota, 2450 Riverside Avenue South, Suite R200,
Minneapolis, MN 55454, USA*
[b]*Gillette Children's Specialty Healthcare Hospital, 200 East University Avenue, St. Paul, MN 55101, USA*
[c]*Shriner's Hospital for Children-Twin Cities Unit, 2025 East River Parkway, Minneapolis, MN 55414, USA*

Wrist deformities occur after fracture because of malunion of the fracture or secondary to injury to the growth plate leading to imbalance of growth. Prevention of malunion is paramount by early recognition with proper reduction and casting or fracture fixation and casting. If a malunions occurs, an osteotomy may be necessary if anticipated growth will not correct the deformity.

Injury of the growth plate may lead to wrist deformity in two ways: angular growth or growth arrest. In the first mechanism, if a portion of the radius or ulna physis is injured, angular growth may result and the bone may grow crooked over time. An example would be a physeal bar leading to angular growth. In the second mechanism, the entire radial or ulnar growth plate is injured, resulting in retardation or arrest of growth. Imbalanced growth between the radius and ulna results in an ulnar-positive or ulnar-negative wrist. Joint leveling is an important concept in wrist deformities after growth plate arrest. A level joint refers to the even growth of the radius and ulna to avoid ulnar impaction (ulnar-positive wrist) or ulnar tethering with radial bowing (ulnar-negative wrist). If considerable growth discrepancy occurs between the ulna and radius, a joint leveling procedure may be necessary. Options include stopping growth in the longer bone, such as an epiphysiodesis or stapling of the physis, or a lengthening or shortening osteotomy

to level the length of the radius and ulna at the wrist.

This article discusses growth plate anatomy and its injuries and wrist deformities that can occur after fracture.

### Growth plate anatomy

Growth of the distal ends of the ulna and radius requires an orderly process through the physis. The physis or growth plate is located between the epiphysis and the metaphysis, as shown in Fig. 1.

The structural organization of the physis allows longitudinal growth of the bone through endochondral ossification. The organization includes the physis located at the end of the metaphyseal bone and the epiphysis at the end of the physis. Physeal growth occurs with stem cells along the epiphyseal border, differentiating into chondrocytes in the more proximal zone [1]. In the more proximal zones, the chondrocytes mature from stages of proliferating to prehypertrophic to hypertrophic chondrocytes. Finally the chondrocyte ossifies into metaphyseal bone [2]. Through this process, the bone is lengthened. The weakest area of the physis is through the zone of hypertrophy and this is the most common line of fracture cleavage [3].

### Growth plate injury

Growth plate injury can occur through disruption of any of the mechanisms that produce normal growth. This can include structural disruption of the physis, so the physis is no longer

* Department of Orthopaedic Surgery, University of Minnesota, 2450 Riverside Avenue South, Suite R200, Minneapolis, MN 55454.
*E-mail address:* vanhe003@umn.edu.

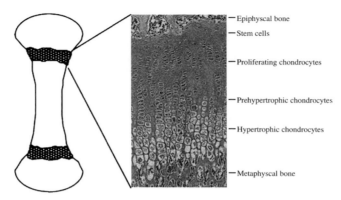

Fig. 1. Growth plate anatomy.

normally aligned. This also can involve physiologic distortion of the physis so that cell damage disrupts normal cellular function.

Growth plate injuries have been classified by Salter and Harris [4]. Different growth disturbances can occur, depending on the type and magnitude of growth plate injury. Growth disturbances commonly include angular growth, growth arrest, or rarely, overgrowth. Metaphyseal fractures also may lead to growth disturbances because of concomitant injury to the nearby growth plate [5,6]. The role of fracture fixation and subsequent growth disturbances is controversial [7,8].

Standard fracture management requires reduction or fixation of displaced growth plate injuries in the first days after injury to obtain anatomic alignment of the physis and to prevent growth disturbances [9]. Distal radius and ulna fractures treated conservatively have been shown to have the worst results in children older than 10 years of age who have more than 20° of angular deformity [10]. Reduction is recommended for children who have more than 20° of angulation and less than 2 years of growth remaining [11].

Fractures involving the distal ulnar physis may be difficult to diagnose because of the late ossification of the distal ulnar physis. Post-traumatic growth arrest of the distal ulnar physis has been reported to be as high as 55% in one series [12]. Traumatic ulnar physeal arrest is associated most commonly with distal radius fractures [13,14]. Premature closure of the distal radial physis after fracture also has been reported [15,16]. In one series [17], growth disturbances after fractures involving the ulnar physis were significantly more common (50%) than after fractures involving the radial physis (4.4%).

Growth plate injury also may occur because of repetitive trauma to the growth plate [18]. Skeletally immature gymnasts have been documented to have an incidence of wrist pain in 56% in one series [19], with 51% showing radiographic evidence of stress injury to the distal radial physis and 7% with frank widening of the growth plate. Factors associated with wrist pain included higher skill level, older age, and more years of training.

## Treatment of wrist deformities

Wrist deformities occur after fracture acutely (because of a malunion of the fracture) or as a late sequela (because of a growth plate injury causing a growth disturbance). Sequelae include angular growth disturbances, growth arrest, or overgrowth.

### Fracture malunions

Osteotomies have been used successfully to treat malunions of the pediatric distal radius [20–23]. Techniques described use internal fixation with plate or pins augmented with possible iliac crest or synthetic bone graft, such as the example shown in Fig. 2.

For fractures of the distal radius or ulna, the major issue is how much deformity can be tolerated and how much remodeling will occur to correct the deformity. One biomechanical study has shown that with radial shortening to any degree, the total contact area in the lunate fossa was increased and was significant at 2 mm of shortening. By angulating the distal radius more than 20° palmar or dorsal, there was a dorsal shift in the scaphoid and lunate high pressure areas,

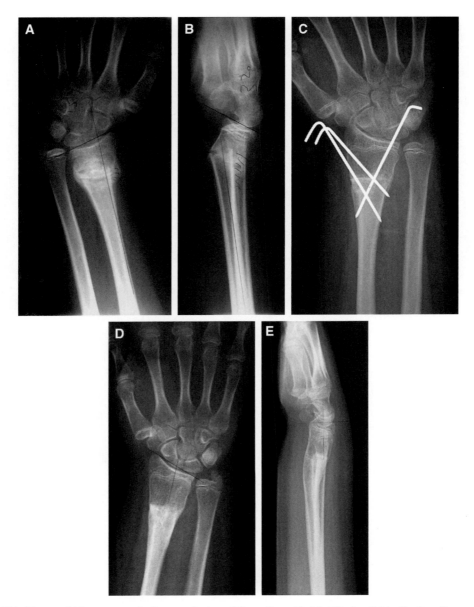

Fig. 2. This 13-year-old boy presented after a malunion of the radius with (*A*) 15° of radial inclination, 2 mm of ulnar-positive variance, and (*B*) 35° of dorsal tilt. (*C*) He was treated with a dorsal opening wedge osteotomy with allograft and pinning. At 1-year follow-up, he was healed (*D* and *E*) with full return to function.

and the loads were more concentrated [24]. Because the normal radial tilt is 11° volar, this biomechanical study indicates that 10° or greater of dorsal radial angulation or 31° or greater of volar angulation is an indication for osteotomy to correct malunions to restore more normal radial–carpal mechanics. Certainly the best treatment

for distal radius or ulnar malunions is prevention with proper initial treatment to achieve anatomic alignment and pin fixation for unstable fractures [25]. Recent recommendations for distal radius fracture reduction and consideration for pin fixation is greater than 25° of sagittal angulation in patients younger than 12 years old and greater

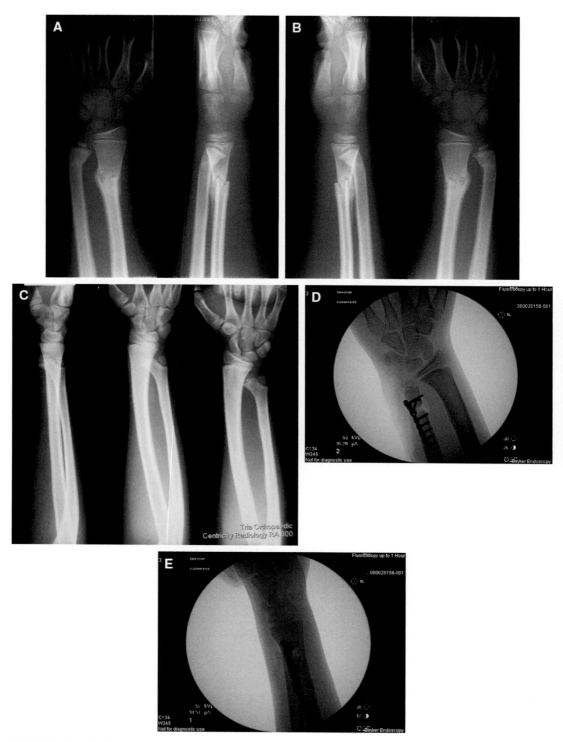

Fig. 3. Distal radial fracture with distal ulnar fracture and physeal injury (*A* and *B*) with angular growth (*C*) treated with excision/osteotomy (*D* and *E*) until union (*F* and *G*). See text for case details.

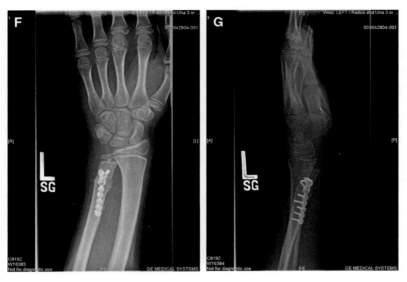

Fig. 3 (*continued*)

than 15° of sagittal angulation or more than 10° of radial deviation in patients older than 12 years old [26]. A healed fracture outside these parameters may be an indication for treatment of the malunion with an osteotomy.

## Angular growth

Angular growth disturbances are corrected most commonly by osteotomy. One example of an angular growth disturbance after a distal ulnar physeal injury is shown in Fig. 3. This 10-year-old boy sustained a distal radius and ulna fracture as shown in Fig. 3A. The distal ulnar physeal injury was not identified at the time of bone union (Fig. 3B). Two years later an angular growth had occurred through the distal ulna, with splitting of the ulnar physis, as shown in Fig. 3C. Although the triangular fibrocartilage complex (TFCC) was shown on MRI to be attached to the more ulnar segment, the more radial segment had a more substantial physeal segment. The ulnar segment was excised and the radial segment was osteotomized with an opening wedge osteotomy to simultaneously correct length, as shown in Figs. 3D,E. The TFCC attachment then was repaired to the radial segment and the osteotomy united (Figs. 3F,G). As demonstrated in this example, osteotomies for angular deformities need to be customized to correct the deformity.

## Overgrowth or growth arrest

In the lower extremity, limb length equality is imperative for normal walking posture. In the upper extremity, limb length equality is less important, because no impairment occurs from minor arm length differences. In the upper extremity, however, length equality of the radius and the ulna is crucial to provide a level joint surface for normal wrist function. A level joint without significant variance between the length of the ulna and the radius leads to more normal wrist function. If a significant growth arrest or overgrowth has occurred as a result of fracture, variance between the length of the ulna and the radius occurs over time, which may impair wrist joint function.

## Ulnar variance

Growth arrest or overgrowth after fracture may lead to significant disparity of length between the radius and the ulna. The average ulnar variance within the general population is between +1.4 mm and −1.8 mm [27]. Depending on the shape of the distal radioulnar joint, some length discrepancy of negative ulnar variance can be accommodated without considerable symptoms, because the distal radioulnar joint in some patients can remodel to accommodate this change. As the length discrepancy increases, however, a short ulna can cause bowing of the radius and ultimately may cause dislocation of the radial head.

How much variance is tolerated before symptoms ensue? A recent study of 163 distal forearm physeal fractures sustained in patients who were 11.6 years old (range, 5–17 years) at the time of injury were followed up at an average of 25.5 years later (range, 14–46 years). At follow-up, all of the patients were fully asymptomatic except for the 10 patients who had forearm bone growth failure of more than 1 cm [17]. At 1 cm of ulnar variance, symptoms were significant and an osteotomy was required. Many patients who had less than 1 cm of ulnar variance may be asymptomatic.

Each patient should be assessed individually by history, inquiring about hand dominance, age and type of previous trauma, and symptoms associated with the wrist deformity; physical examination should include range of motion, grip strength, and pain with pronation, supination, radial deviation, and ulnar deviation (ulnar impaction test); wrist radiographs include a PA of the wrist in neutral rotation with the elbow at 90° of flexion to assess properly for ulnar variance.

### Ulnar-positive variance

Ulnar-positive variance is usually more symptomatic than ulnar-negative variance. Ulnar-positive variance is caused by overgrowth of the ulna

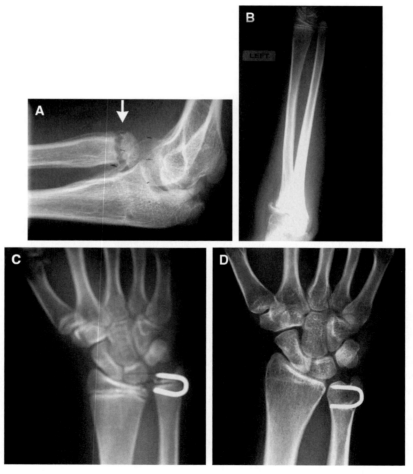

Fig. 4. This radial neck fracture (*A*) led to complete growth arrest of the proximal radius and resultant proximal migration of the radius and ulnar impaction at the wrist (*B*). Stapling of the distal ulnar epiphysiodesis (*C*) allowed growth to level the joint over 4 years until the patient was skeletally mature (*D*).

or growth arrest of the radius. Most patients present with pain and limited range of motion. The diagnosis of ulnar impaction syndrome can be confirmed on physical examination with pain elicited on ulnar deviation and compression.

Treatment of symptomatic discrepancies in ulnar variance is a joint-leveling procedure. The length discrepancy between the ulna and the radius can be corrected by several methods [28]. In the growing child or early adolescent, the growth in the longer bone can be halted by epiphysiodesis or stapling of the physis. The growth remaining can be estimated by looking at age, skeletal maturity of the contralateral unaffected limb, length of their same gender parent's limb, or by consulting growth remaining graphs [29]. A case example of a wrist deformity after a radial head fracture with a complete growth arrest of the proximal radius is shown in Fig. 4A. With a positive ulnar variance of 10 mm at age 12 years (Fig. 4B), a stapling was performed of the distal ulna. With continued growth over the next 4 years, the final ulnar variance was 1 mm (Figs. 4C,D). The staple was asymptomatic and was left in place. This is an example of slowing the growth in the longer bone to level the joint over time.

If the wrist is symptomatic because of ulnar impaction after skeletal maturity, a lengthening or shortening osteotomy can be recommended to achieve a level joint. Most commonly after fracture the length discrepancy between the radius and ulna would be modest (less than 2 cm). With less than 2 cm of discrepancy, an acute ulnar shortening osteotomy would be the most practical joint leveling procedure, as shown in Fig. 5. Shortening osteotomy techniques of the ulna [30] include step-cut osteotomy, a resection osteotomy, and an oblique osteotomy [31] as shown in Fig. 5.

### Ulnar-negative variance

Most commonly, with severe negative ulnar variance, a lengthening osteotomy of the ulna would be recommended. This type of severe negative ulnar variance occurs more commonly because of multiple hereditary exostoses with significant impairment of distal ulnar physeal growth, although it can be seen after fracture or infection of the distal ulnar physis. The techniques for lengthening include distraction osteogenesis of the ulna [32] and acute ulnar lengthening osteotomy [33]. Alternatively an epiphysiodesis or stapling of the distal radius in the child who has growth remaining could be considered. If an osteotomy is performed in a child who has growth remaining, it may need to be repeated at skeletal maturity to level the joint.

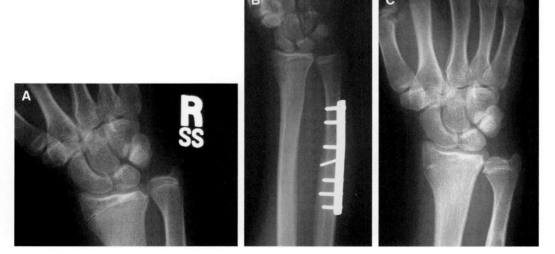

Fig. 5. This 13-year-old girl elite level junior tennis player presented with a longstanding painful wrist in her dominant hand. Ulnar impaction syndrome secondary to premature radial physeal closure was diagnosed (*A*) and treated with a precision oblique osteotomy and plating (*B*). The patient went on to union (*C*) and was asymptomatic but was not able to return to elite level tennis.

## References

[1] Iannotti JP. Growth plate physiology and pathology. Orthop Clin North Am 1990;21(1):1–17.

[2] van der Eerden BC, Karperien M, Wit JM. Systemic and local regulation of the growth plate. Endocr Rev 2003;24(6):782–801.

[3] Jones E. Growth and development as related to trauma. In: Green NE, Swiontkowski M, editors. Skeletal trauma in children. 2nd edition. Vol. 3. Philadelphia, PA: WB Saunders; 1998. p. 1–15.

[4] Salter RB, Harris WR. Injuries involving the epiphyseal plate. Inst Course Lect. J Bone Joint Surg [Am] 1963;45-A(3):587–622.

[5] Williams AA, Szabo RM. Case report: radial overgrowth and deformity after metaphyseal fracture fixation in a child. Clin Orthop Relat Res 2005; 435:258–62.

[6] Tang CW, Kay RM, Skaggs DL. Growth arrest of the distal radius following a metaphyseal fracture: case report and review of the literature. J Pediatr Orthop [Br] 2002;11(1):89–92.

[7] Flynn JM, Sarwark JF, Waters PM, et al. The surgical management of pediatric fractures of the upper extremity. Instr Course Lect 2003;52:635–45.

[8] Pritchett JW. Does pinning cause distal radial growth plate arrest? Orthopaedics 1994;17(6):550–2.

[9] Dicke TE, Nunley JA. Distal forearm fractures in children. Complications and surgical indications. Orthop Clin North Am 1993;24(2):333–40.

[10] Zimmermann R, Gschwentner M, Kralinger F, et al. Long-term results following pediatric distal forearm fractures. Arch Orthop Trauma Surg 2004;124(3): 179–86.

[11] Noonan KJ, Price CT. Forearm and distal radius fractures in children. J Am Acad Orthop Surg 1998;6(3):146–56.

[12] Golz RJ, Grogan DP, Greene TL, et al. Distal ulnar physeal injury. J Pediatr Orthop 1991;11(3):318–26.

[13] Ray TD, Tessler RH, Dell PC. Traumatic ulnar physeal arrest after distal forearm fractures in children. J Pediatr Orthop 1996;16(2):195–200.

[14] Nelson OA, Buchanan JR, Harrison CS. Distal ulnar growth arrest. J Hand Surg [Am] 1984;9(2): 164–70.

[15] Valverde JA, Albinana J, Certucha JA. Early posttraumatic physeal arrest in distal radius after a compression injury. J Pediatr Orthop B 1996;5(1): 57–60.

[16] Hernandez J Jr, Peterson HA. Fracture of the distal radial physis complicated by compartment syndrome and premature physeal closure. J Pediatr Orthop 1986;6(5):627–30.

[17] Cannata G, De Maio F, Mancini F, et al. Physeal fractures of the distal radius and ulna: long-term prognosis. J Orthop Trauma 2003;17(3):172–9; discussion 179–80.

[18] Liebling MS, Berdon WE, Ruzal-Shapiro C, et al. Gymnast's wrist (pseudorickets growth plate abnormality) in adolescent athletes: findings on plain films and MR imaging. Am J Roentgenol 1995;164(1): 157–9.

[19] DiFiori JP, Puffer JC, Aish B, et al. Wrist pain, distal radial physeal injury, and ulnar variance in young gymnasts: does a relationship exist? Am J Sports Med 2002;30(6):879–85.

[20] Meier R, Prommersberger KJ, van Griensven M, et al. Surgical correction of deformities of the distal radius due to fractures in pediatric patients. Arch Orthop Trauma Surg 2004;124(1):1–9.

[21] Friberg KS. Remodelling after distal forearm fractures in children. III. Correction of residual angulation in fractures of the radius. Acta Orthop Scand 1979;50(6 Pt 2):741–9.

[22] Hove LM, Engesaeter LB. Corrective osteotomies after injuries of the distal radial physis in children. J Hand Surg [Br] 1997;22(6):699–704.

[23] Zehntner MK, Jakob RP, McGanity PL. Growth disturbance of the distal radial epiphysis after trauma: operative treatment by corrective radial osteotomy. J Pediatr Orthop 1990;10(3):411–5.

[24] Pogue DJ, Viegas SF, Patterson RM, et al. Effects of distal radius fracture malunion on wrist joint mechanics. J Hand Surg [Am] 1990;15(5):721–7.

[25] Gibbons CL, Woods DA, Pailthorpe C, et al. The management of isolated distal radius fractures in children. J Pediatr Orthop 1994;14(2):207–10.

[26] Flynn JM, Sarwark JF, Waters PM, et al. The operative management of pediatric fractures of the upper extremity. J Bone Joint Surg [Am] 2002;84(11): 2078–89.

[27] Freedman DM, Edwards GS Jr, Willems MJ, et al. Right versus left symmetry of ulnar variance. A radiographic assessment. Clin Orthop Relat Res 1998;354:153–8.

[28] Waters PM, Bae DS, Montgomery KD. Surgical management of posttraumatic distal radial growth arrest in adolescents. J Pediatr Orthop 2002;22(6): 717–24.

[29] Bortel DT, Pritchett JW. Straight-line graphs for the prediction of growth of the upper extremities. J Bone Joint Surg [Am] 1993;75(6):885–92.

[30] Lee BS, Esterhai JL Jr, Das M. Fracture of the distal radial epiphysis. Characteristics and surgical treatment of premature, post-traumatic epiphyseal closure. Clin Orthop Relat Res 1984;185:90–6.

[31] Rayhack JM, Gasser SI, Latta LL, et al. Precision oblique osteotomy for shortening of the ulna. J Hand Surg [Am] 1993;18(5):908–18.

[32] Abe M, Shirai H, Okamoto M, et al. Lengthening of the forearm by callus distraction. J Hand Surg [Br] 1996;21(2):151–63.

[33] Waters PM, Van Heest AE, Emans J. Acute forearm lengthenings. J Pediatr Orthop 1997;17(4):444–9.

ELSEVIER
SAUNDERS

Hand Clin 22 (2006) 121–129

HAND
CLINICS

# Elbow Deformities After Fracture

Shawn W. Storm, DO[a], D. Patrick Williams, DO[a],
Joseph Khoury, MD[b], John D. Lubahn, MD[a],*

[a]*Hamot Medical Center, Hand, Microsurgery and Reconstructive Orthopaedics,
300 State Street, Suite 205, Erie, PA 16507, USA*
[b]*Shriners Hospitals for Children, 1645 W. 8th Street, Erie, PA 16505, USA*

Angular deformities of the distal humerus are a common complication after elbow fracture in children. Cubitus varus (gunstock deformity) Fig. 1 is the most common deformity following supracondylar fracture of the humerus. The average reported incidence after supracondylar fracture is 30%, ranging from 0% to 60% reported in the literature [1]. The usual etiology of the deformity is malreduction and malunion of the fracture rather than growth arrest [2]. The deformity occurs as a result of residual coronal angulation (varus tilt) that is aggravated by malrotation and hyperextension [3].

Historically patients who have residual cubitus varus deformity have little functional disability. Labele and colleagues [1] performed a retrospective study of 63 patients who had cubitus varus following supracondylar fracture of the humerus. The investigators found no functional differences between those who underwent corrective osteotomy and those who were simply observed. They also concluded that the indications for osteotomy were merely cosmetic. They emphasized the need to clarify this notion with patients preoperatively because of the high complication rate associated with operative intervention. Complication rates after surgery average roughly 20% [4] with some sources reporting rates as high as 33% [1]. Other studies, however, suggest that cubitus varus is more than just an issue of cosmesis. Long-term studies have demonstrated that there can be a high incidence of tardy ulnar nerve palsy after

cubitus varus deformity [5]. Davids and colleagues [6] demonstrated an increased risk for fracture of the lateral humeral condyle in patients who have cubitus varus. Impairment in throwing athletes also has been reported [3].

### Deformity analysis and osteotomy planning

Deformity analysis and osteotomy planning considerations are similar to those in the lower extremity. First the deformity needs to be characterized accurately in all three planes. In the coronal plane, Baumann's angle can be used, but a radiographic carrying angle compared with the other side is simpler to use and works well. In the sagittal plane, numerous radiographic measurement techniques exist; however, in a chronic deformity, the clinical assessment of flexion contracture or hyperextension deformity is more practical and must be taken into consideration when planning the osteotomy. As described by Kim [7], the clinician can be misled easily when assessing sagittal plane deformity. He stresses the importance of manually maintaining the epicondylar axis parallel to the floor when making sagittal plane assessment. Finally, axial deformity is an often overlooked yet extremely important component of the deformity. Usually a clinical assessment made in comparison with the opposite limb is sufficient, but if the other components of the deformity are severe, a CT scan including shoulder and elbow may be needed.

Once the deformity has been characterized clearly in all three planes, the planning stage begins. The important thing to realize is that the true deformity is close to the joint, whereas the

* Corresponding author.
*E-mail address:* jdlubahn@adelphia.net
(J.D. Lubahn).

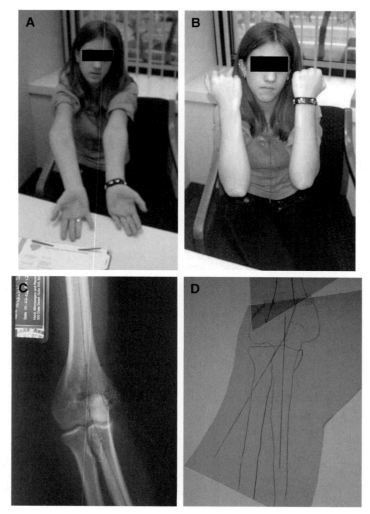

Fig. 1. (*A* and *B*) Clinical alignment of the elbow in a 14-year-old girl who had cubitus varus. She has full flexion and extension preoperatively, but a significant gunstock deformity. (*C*) Radiographs of the same patient. Cubitus varus is secondary to a supracondylar fracture treated initially with closed reduction and percutaneous K-wire fixation. The patient is left with 15° of residual varus. (*D*) Template outlined from the radiograph shown in (*C*) before the osteotomy of the humerus. Templates are crucial in the preoperative planning process. (*E*) Intraoperative radiograph of the same patient after osteotomy performed as a locking step cut and held with crossed K-wires stabilized with cross K-wires. (*F*) Radiograph 1 year after osteotomy showing complete correction with excellent radiographic alignment of the distal humerus and correction of the cubitus varus. (*G* and *H*) The same patient 2 years after osteotomy, demonstrating full flexion and extension of her elbows. She is a cheerleader for a local high school and is able to participate in pyramids, catch other cheerleaders tossed in the air, and most recently, perform a back handspring.

correction is planned at some level proximal to the joint. Any standard angular correction technique (opening or closing wedge) therefore results in a secondary translational deformity in the distal fragment. Because of the subcutaneous anatomy of the elbow, even mild translation can be cosmetically unacceptable. With this in mind, a dome type of osteotomy or rotational step cut as described by Kim [7] moves the axis of correction closer to the deformity, which minimizes secondary translation. These osteotomies generally are planned in the coronal plane (on the AP radiograph). After the cuts are made, flexion/extension correction can be added with little additional

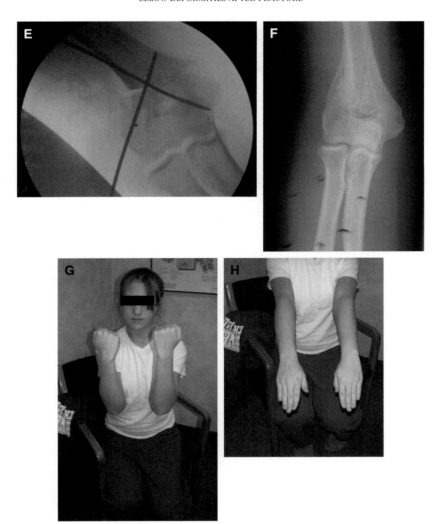

Fig. 1 (*continued*)

work. Incorporating major rotational correction adds major complexity to the planning. Moderate amounts of rotation can be corrected with the dome, but major correction may require the use of gradual distraction. With all techniques and implants the osteotomy should be planned so that the axis of correction is as close to the deformity as possible.

## Cubitus varus

Controversy exists in the treatment of angular malalignment after supracondylar fractures. Options include observation, hemiepiphysiodesis,

and osteotomy. Observation has little role in the treatment of varus malalignment. Little growth occurs at the physis about the elbow, therefore there is little remodeling potential. Some remodeling potential may exist in the younger child if the deformity lies within the plane of motion of the joint (ie, hyperextension). In the older child, however, there is little remodeling potential even in the plane of motion of the joint [2].

Hemiepiphysiodesis may be of benefit in the setting of medial growth arrest or trochlear avascular necrosis. Without treatment medial growth arrest leads to progressive worsening varus deformity secondary to lateral overgrowth.

Hemiepiphysiodesis, however, is not indicated in the much more common setting of varus malreduction with a normal physis [2]. Corrective osteotomy is the only treatment to truly address the angular deformity of cubitus varus.

Multiple osteotomies of varied complexity have been reported in the literature to achieve correction of post-traumatic cubitus varus. Each osteotomy technique has its inherent advantages and limitations. The three most popular techniques are the lateral closing wedge osteotomy (LCWO) (Fig. 1B), the step cut LCWO, and the dome rotational osteotomy. The osteotomy performed most commonly is the lateral closing wedge osteotomy as first described by Siris in 1939 [8]. There have been several modifications to the original procedure with mixed results [9]. Ippolito and colleagues [9] have reported on the long-term follow-up LCWO with 50% poor results related to loss of correction and recurrence of deformity. Although the LCWO is technically a safe and simple procedure, there are many problems associated with it. The lateral scar oftentimes can become hypertrophic. Other shortcomings include inadequate secure fixation and difficulty achieving secure fixation [10]. Furthermore there is a tendency toward a prominence of the lateral condyle, which may compromise final cosmetic outcome [3].

DeRosa and Graziano [11] described an interlocking step cut LCWO secured with a single screw. (The authors also have used cross K-wires.) They reported good and excellent results in 10 of 11 patients. Their one poor result was in a patient who had residual varus secondary to an unrecognized fracture of the cortical spike. The advantage to the step cut LCWO is the added stability of the osteotomy. The main shortcoming associated with this technique is the limited medial and lateral translation of the distal fragment [11]. Moreover the distal fragment can be rotated only in the horizontal plane to correct the deformity.

The dome rotational osteotomy was popularized in Japan [12] (R. Kanaujia, I. Yoshikazu, H. Muneshige, unpublished data). Advantages of the dome osteotomy are that it can reorient the distal fragment in the coronal and horizontal planes. There is therefore less residual prominence of the lateral condyle associated with this osteotomy. Rotation in the coronal plane may be limited or difficult to achieve, however, secondary to medial soft tissue contracture [9]. Kanaujia and coworkers [13] published a 5-year follow-up in 11 children who had varus deformity after

supracondylar fracture treated with dome osteotomy. The investigators report satisfactory results in all 11 patients with respect to deformity correction and complication rate. Other techniques for correction of cubitus varus have been proposed.

King and Secor [14] described a medial opening wedge osteotomy (MOWO), which has the advantages of maintaining humeral length and better cosmesis through a medially-based incision. In addition, the osteotomy does not produce a secondary translational deformity. The disadvantage stems from lengthening the medial structures, which may result in an ulnar neuropraxia [14]. Moreover, MOWOs take longer to heal and therefore require long-term cast immobilization, which is not desirable in adolescents and adults. Laupattarakasem and colleagues [15] described a pentagonal ("pentalateral") osteotomy with 88% good or excellent results in 58 patients with 16-month follow-up. A satisfactory carrying angle was obtained in all cases without complications. This technique avoids the prominence of the lateral condyle but is technically challenging and difficult to perform consistently. In general, as the complexity of the osteotomy increases, so does the complication rate.

## Lateral condyle fractures

Fractures of the lateral humeral condyle are the second most common fracture about the elbow in children after supracondylar fractures, with an incidence of 1.6 in 10,000 [16] (Fig. 2A). They represent serious injury and the management of lateral condylar fractures is fraught with complications. One of the most common complications secondary to lateral humeral condyle fractures is, in fact, cubitus valgus. Wilkins [3] classified problems affecting treatment outcome after lateral condylar fractures into two broad categories: (1) biologic (problems associated with the healing process) and (2) technical (errors in management). Biologic-related problems include lateral condylar spur formation (overgrowth) and cubitus varus. Technical-related problems include nonunion, cubitus valgus, and avascular necrosis.

Lateral condylar spur formation results from overgrowth of the periosteal flap that is avulsed from the proximal fragment [3]. The prominence may give the appearance of cubitus varus (pseudovarus). The overgrowth, however, usually remodels and eventually disappears. There is seldom a cosmetic or functional problem with spur

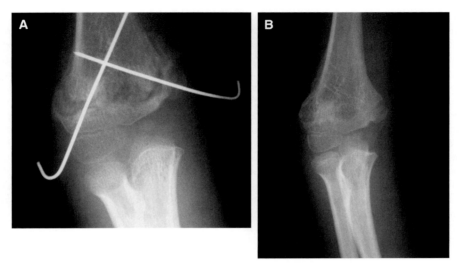

Fig. 2. (*A*) Represents a cross-pinning of a lateral condyle fracture with concomitant supracondylar fracture. (*B*) Cubitus varus secondary to a lateral condyle fracture.

formation, so treatment should consist of reassurance and observation.

Cubitus varus occurs in as many as 42% of lateral condyle fractures [17,18] (Fig. 2B). Although the cause of the deformity is not entirely understood, it is believed to be secondary to a combination of lateral condylar physeal stimulation or inadequate reduction [2]. Despite the high incidence of deformity, cubitus varus usually is mild and rarely is severe enough to cause concern or warrant surgical correction. Some investigators have reported that children who have cubitus varus have pain, decreased range of motion, epicondylitis, and interference with sporting activities [2]. Davids and coworkers reported an increased risk for lateral condyle fracture in patients who have post-traumatic cubitus varus [6]. They concluded that cubitus varus is more than just a cosmetic deformity, advocating a two-stage correction of the deformity (first anatomic reduction and internal fixation of the lateral condyle followed by valgus supracondylar osteotomy).

Nonunion of lateral humeral condyle fractures is believed to be a technical complication. Flynn and colleagues [19] established criteria for nonunion if the fracture had not united by 12 weeks. Nonunion of lateral condyle fractures can result in progressive cubitus valgus deformity [20–22] and tardy ulnar nerve palsy [20,22–24]. The treatment of established nonunion of the lateral condyle is controversial and laden with complications [25–29]. Some investigators advocate nonoperative

treatment in established nonunions of the lateral condyle, citing loss of range of motion and avascular necrosis postoperatively as reasons not to operate [25,30–32]. Many patients who have established long-term nonunion have no functional disability and only cosmetic deformity, adding further support for nonoperative treatment [5,33,34]. Flynn and Richards [19] and others [18,27,32,35], however, have obtained satisfactory results in treating lateral condyle nonunion. Flynn recognized the important distinction between a nonunion in good position and one in poor position. He advocated early surgery for established nonunion when the condylar fragment is in good position. If, however, the condylar fragment is in poor position, he advised against surgery because of the high likelihood of damage to the physeal plate of the fragment and subsequent growth arrest leading to valgus deformity [19].

In patients who have a simple, more recent nonunion and minimal displacement, compressive screws across the metaphyseal portion is all that is usually necessary. Bone grafting seldom is needed in such cases. In established nonunions the fracture site needs to be explored and the nonunion taken down so as to provide fresh cancellous surfaces for opposition [3]. Supplemental bone grafting may be required if a significant gap exists. Moreover, the fixation must provide compression across the fracture site and provide enough stability to allow early active range of motion. Patients must be cautioned about potential loss of elbow motion. Usually this loss of motion (extension) is 10° to 15° and does not interfere with functional capabilities; however, some have reported losses as high as 60% [36].

Delayed open reduction is problematic and controversy exists as to whether elbow function can be improved by doing a late open reduction and internal fixation. The rationale for treating late lateral condyle fractures is to obtain union and prevent cubitus valgus, tardy ulnar nerve palsy, pain, and instability. There have been many reports in the literature of avascular necrosis after late reduction [25,32,37]. This has been attributed to the extensive soft tissue stripping and subsequent devascularization associated with trying to achieve an accurate anatomic reduction [19]. Jakob and Fowles [25] reported on delayed surgery and found that those patients treated later than 3 weeks after fracture did no better than those who received no treatment at all. Furthermore, the surgical patients lost on average 34° range of motion, and there was a high incidence of avascular necrosis, premature physeal closure, and valgus deformity. They concluded avascular necrosis is iatrogenic and most often occurs in cases treated late or in nonunions and delayed unions. Roye and colleagues [29] reported good results in the late surgical treatment of lateral condylar fracture in four children 8 weeks to 14 years after injury. They stress the importance of avoiding posterior dissection to maintain blood supply to the fracture fragment. More recently, Shimada and colleagues [38] reported good to excellent results in 15 of 16 patients at an average follow-up of 11 years after osteosynthesis for nonunion of fractures of the lateral condyle. The one patient who had a poor result had evidence of avascular necrosis. Wattenbarger and colleagues [39] reported no cases of avascular necrosis in 11 patients treated with late (>3 weeks) open reduction internal fixation of lateral condyle fractures. In this series, imperfect reductions were accepted in lieu of extensive posterior dissection. Despite a lack of anatomic reduction, all patients had good to excellent results with near full range of motion, an acceptable carrying angle, and little or no pain at an average of 6.3 years' follow-up.

The most common sequela of lateral condyle nonunion with displacement is the development of a progressive cubitus valgus deformity [2]. Cubitus valgus occurs from nonunion and proximal migration of the lateral condyle, not from premature closure of the capitellar physis. Nonsurgical treatment is appropriate for asymptomatic nonunion of the lateral condyle. Patients who have asymptomatic nonunion, cubitus valgus, and tardy ulnar nerve palsy should be treated with ulnar nerve transposition [2]. The treatment of established nonunion of the lateral condyle in symptomatic patients who have cubitus valgus is controversial. Surgery is not always successful and frequently leads to loss of motion even when successful. Recently Kim and colleagues [7] achieved union in only 2 of 4 patients who had an established nonunion of the lateral condyle and cubitus valgus deformity.

Tardy ulnar nerve palsy is a well-known late complication of fractures of the lateral condyle. In 1924 Miller [40] noted 47% of his patients who had tardy ulnar nerve palsy had a fracture of the lateral condylar physis as a child. The onset of symptoms was gradual and varied from 30 to 40 years. In Gay and Love's [23] series of 100 patients, the average interval of onset was 22 years. Motor loss occurred first, followed by sensory changes. Various methods of treatment have been advocated, ranging from anterior transposition of the ulnar nerve to simple release of the cubital tunnel.

## Fishtail deformity

Fishtail deformity of the distal humerus as coined by Wilson [41] in 1955 is an uncommon complication seen after fracture of the lateral condylar physis (Fig. 3A). The deformity may be the result of any one of three different causes according to Nwakama and colleagues [42]. Premature growth arrest of the mid-portion of the distal humeral physis is one potential cause; another is failure to anatomically reduce an intercondylar fracture of the distal humerus, leaving a gap in reduction in the intercondylar notch. Finally, avascular necrosis of the trochlea, beginning on the medial side of the elbow and often involving the entire trochlea, is another possible explanation. With continued growth of the lateral or medial physis, a sharp, wedge-shaped intercondylar notch is produced that may impinge the proximal ulna and lead to diminished elbow motion [42]. Wilkins [2] described two types of fishtail deformity. The first type involves the lateral portion of the medial crista at the apex of the trochlea and is seen most commonly after distal supracondylar fractures and lateral condylar fractures. The second type involves the entire trochlea and often some portion of the medial metaphysis. It may be seen after separation of the entire distal humeral epiphysis in older

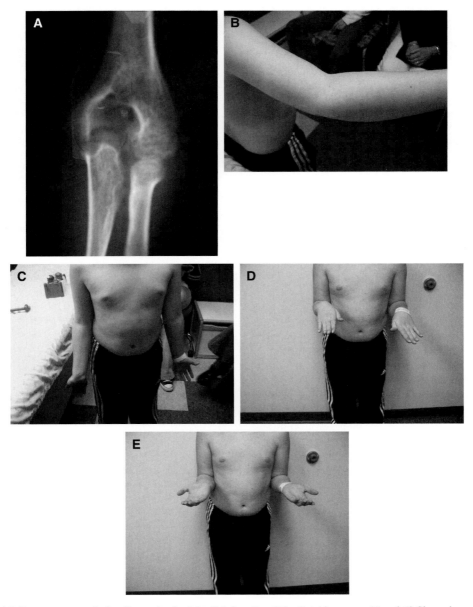

Fig. 3. (*A*) Represents a typical radiograph of a fishtail deformity of the distal humerus. (*B* and *C*) Shows loss of extension secondary to distal humerus fishtail deformity. (*D* and *E*) Shows full supination and pronation despite the distal humerus fishtail deformity.

children or in medial condylar fractures [42]. The development of the distal humerus in the growing child is fairly predictable in that the capitellum begins to ossify at 1 year of age. The trochlea may not appear until the age of 9 years and usually develops with multiple ossific nuclei. The blood supply to the distal end of the humerus is described by Haraldsson [43]. Injection studies show the trochlea is supplied by one or two small end arteries. La-Grange and Rigault [44] and Yang [45] have confirmed these studies showing that the distal end of the growing humerus is supplied by blood vessels that enter the bone at the attachment of the flexor and the extensor muscles.

The general perception among orthopedists is that the fishtail deformity is of little significance. Peterson and coworkers [42], however, noted grave functional disability in three patients because of premature degenerative arthrosis of the elbow. Moreover, they uncovered another potential late complication: intercondylar fracture predisposed by the altered mechanics of the distal humerus. In fact, the shape of the fishtail may vary from patient to patient depending on the location and extent of the injury to the trochlea, capitellum, or central distal humeral epiphysis (Fig. 3B–E).

No uniformly effective primary treatment is known for avascular necrosis of the distal humeral epiphysis. Once the partial physeal arrest is noted, attempts to minimize the ensuing deformity should be considered. Surgical arrest of the remaining lateral or medial physis may be given consideration. The humeral length discrepancy would not be any greater than that produced by the central arrest. Moreover, the distal humerus only accounts for 15% of humeral longitudinal growth and therefore would not cause a functional length problem. Troublesome residual angular deformity can be corrected by osteotomy [42].

## Summary

Nonunion of the lateral humeral condyle, cubitus varus, cubitus valgus, and fishtail deformity represent particularly challenging problems to the upper extremity surgeon. Although closed or open reduction and pinning of supracondylar fractures of the distal humerus can restore anatomic alignment and avoid anatomic deformities in most cases, closed reduction is still a common form of treatment. In those hopefully few cases in which reduction is less than optimal, or when a good reduction is performed but subsequently lost between follow-up visits, the aforementioned deformities of the distal humerus can develop. Even when anatomic reduction is obtained and held, avascular necrosis of the trochlea may develop, leading to the so-called fishtail deformity. Although not recognized for several years, and when initially recognized, not necessarily taken seriously, fishtail deformity may be one of the more devastating deformities in that it is not correctable by traditional methods of osteotomy. Flexion contracture when present may be treated by standard release; however, when a bony block exists as a result of the shape of the fishtail, no surgical options exist and the patient often is left with a permanent loss of motion.

## References

[1] Labelle H, Bunnell WP, Duhaime M, et al. Cubitus varus deformity following supracondylar fractures of the humerus in children. J Pediatr Orthop 1982; 2(5):539–46.

[2] Wilkins K. Fractures and dislocations of the elbow region. In: Rockwood C, Wilkins K, King RE, editors. Fractures in children. 4th edition. Vol. 3. Philadelphia: Lippincott-Raven; 1996. p. 363–575.

[3] Wilkins KE. Residuals of elbow trauma in children. Orthop Clin North Am 1990;21(2):291–314.

[4] Voss FR, Kasser JR, Trepman E, et al. Uniplanar supracondylar humeral osteotomy with preset Kirschner wires for posttraumatic cubitus varus. J Pediatr Orthop 1994;14(4):471–8.

[5] Smith FM. An eighty-four year follow-up on a patient with ununited fracture of the lateral condyle of the humerus. A case report. J Bone Joint Surg 1973;55A(2):378–80.

[6] Davids JR, Maguire MF, Mubarak SJ, et al. Lateral condylar fracture of the humerus following post-traumatic cubitus varus. J Pediatr Orthop 1994; 14(4):466–70.

[7] Kim HT, Lee JS, Yoo CI. Management of cubitus varus and valgus. J Bone Joint Surg 2005;87A(4): 771–80.

[8] Smith L. Deformity following supracondylar fractures of the humerus. Am J Orthop 1960;42A: 235–52.

[9] Ippolito E, Moneta MR, D'Arrigo C. Post-traumatic cubitus varus. Long-term follow-up of corrective supracondylar humeral osteotomy in children. J Bone Joint Surg 1990;72A(5):757–65.

[10] Uchida Y, Ogata K, Sugioka Y. A new three-dimensional osteotomy for cubitus varus deformity after supracondylar fracture of the humerus in children. J Pediatr Orthop 1991;11(3):327–31.

[11] DeRosa GP, Graziano GP. A new osteotomy for cubitus varus. Clin Orthop 1988;236:160–5.

[12] Higaki T, Ikuta Y. The new operation method of the domed osteotomy for 4 children with varus deformity of the elbow joint. J Jap Orthop 1982;31: 30–5.

[13] Kanaujia RR, Ikuta Y, Muneshige H, et al. Dome osteotomy for cubitus varus in children. Acta Orthop Scand 1988;59(3):314–7.

[14] King D, Secor C. Bow elbow (cubitus varus). J Bone Joint Surg 1951;33A(3):572–6.

[15] Laupattarakasem W, Mahaisavariya B, Kowsuwon W, et al. Pentalateral osteotomy for cubitus varus. Clinical experiences of a new technique. J Bone Joint Surg 1989;71B(4):667–70.

[16] Landin LA, Danielsson LG. Elbow fractures in children. An epidemiological analysis of 589 cases. Acta Orthop Scand 1986;57(4):309–12.

[17] So YC, Fang D, Leong JC, et al. Varus deformity following lateral humeral condylar fractures in children. J Pediatr Orthop 1985;5(5):569–72.

[18] Foster DE, Sullivan JA, Gross RH. Lateral humeral condylar fractures in children. J Pediatr Orthop 1985;5(1):16–22.

[19] Flynn JC, Richards JF Jr, Saltzman RI. Prevention and treatment of non-union of slightly displaced fractures of the lateral humeral condyle in children. An end-result study. J Bone Joint Surg 1975; 57A(8):1087–92.

[20] Toh S, Tsubo K, Nishikawa S, et al. Long-standing nonunion of fractures of the lateral humeral condyle. J Bone Joint Surg 2002;84A(4):593–8.

[21] Holst-Nielsen F, Ottsen P. Fractures of the lateral condyle of the humerus in children. Acta Orthop Scand 1974;45(4):518–28.

[22] Tien YC, Chen JC, Fu YC, et al. Supracondylar dome osteotomy for cubitus valgus deformity associated with a lateral condylar nonunion in children. J Bone Joint Surg 2005;87(7):1456–63.

[23] Gay J, Love J. Diagnosis and treatment of tardy paralysis of the ulnar nerve: a study of 100 cases. J Bone Joint Surg 1947;29:1087–97.

[24] McGowan AJ. The results of transposition of the ulnar nerve for traumatic ulnar neuritis. J Bone Joint Surg 1950;32B(3):293–301.

[25] Jakob R, Fowles JV, Rang M, et al. Observations concerning fractures of the lateral humeral condyle in children. J Bone Joint Surg 1975;57B(4):430–6.

[26] Devito D, Blackstock S, Minkowitz B. Nonoperative treatment of lateral condyle elbow fractures in children. Miami: POSNA; 1995.

[27] Finnbogason T, Karlsson G, Lindberg L, et al. Nondisplaced and minimally displaced fractures of the lateral humeral condyle in children: a prospective radiographic investigation of fracture stability. J Pediatr Orthop 1995;15(4):422–5.

[28] Mintzer C, Waters PM. Acute open reduction of a displaced scaphoid fracture in a child. J Hand Surg 1994;19A(5):760–1.

[29] Roye DP Jr, Bini SA, Infosino A. Late surgical treatment of lateral condylar fractures in children. J Pediatr Orthop 1991;11(2):195–9.

[30] Toh S, Tsubo K, Nishikawa S, et al. Osteosynthesis for nonunion of the lateral humeral condyle. Clin Orthop 2002;405:230–41.

[31] Fontanetta P, Mackenzie DA, Rosman M. Missed, maluniting, and malunited fractures of the lateral humeral condyle. J Trauma 1978;18(5): 329–35.

[32] Hardacre JA, Nahigian SH, Froimson AI, et al. Fractures of the lateral condyle of the humerus in children. J Bone Joint Surg 1971;53A(6):1083–95.

[33] Moorhead E. Old untreated fracture of external condyle of humerus: factors influencing choice of treatment. Surg Clin 1919;3:987–9.

[34] Morgan SJ, Beaver WB. Nonunion of a pediatric lateral condyle fracture without ulnar nerve palsy: sixty-year follow-up. J Orthop Trauma 1999;13(6):456–8.

[35] Flynn JC. Nonunion of slightly displaced fractures of the lateral humeral condyle in children: an update. J Pediatr Orthop 1989;9(6):691–6.

[36] Masada K, Kawai H, Kawabata H, et al. Osteosynthesis for old, established non-union of the lateral condyle of the humerus. J Bone Joint Surg 1990; 72A(1):32–40.

[37] Dhillon KS, Sengupta S, Singh BJ. Delayed management of fracture of the lateral humeral condyle in children. Acta Orthop Scand 1988;59(4):419–24.

[38] Shimada K, Masada K, Tada K, et al. Osteosynthesis for the treatment of non-union of the lateral humeral condyle in children. J Bone Joint Surg 1997; 79A(2):234–40.

[39] Wattenbarger JM, Gerardi J, Johnston CE. Late open reduction internal fixation of lateral condyle fractures. J Pediatr Orthop 2002;22(3):394–8.

[40] Miller E. Late ulnar nerve palsy. Surg Gynecol Obstet 1924;38:37–46.

[41] Wilson JN. Fractures of the external condyle of the humerus in children. Br J Surg 1955;43(177):88–94.

[42] Nwakama AC, Peterson HA, Shaughnessy WJ. Fishtail deformity following fracture of the distal humerus in children: historical review, case presentations, discussion of etiology, and thoughts on treatment. J Pediatric Orthop Part B 2000;9(4): 309–18.

[43] Haraldsson S. On osteochondrosis deformans juvenilis capituli humeri including investigation of intra-osseous vasculature in distal humerus. Acta Orthop Scand 1959;(Suppl 38):1–232.

[44] LaGrange J, Rigault P. Les fractures de l'extremite inferieure de l'humerus chez l'enfant. II. Fractures du condyle extreme. [French] Rev Clin Orthop 1962;48:415–46.

[45] Yang Z, Wang Y, Gilula LA, et al. Microcirculation of the distal humeral epiphyseal cartilage: implications for post-traumatic growth deformities. J Hand Surg 1998;23A(1):165–72.

**ELSEVIER
SAUNDERS**

Hand Clin 22 (2006) 131

**HAND
CLINICS**

# Erratum

Please note that in the August 2005 issue of *Hand Clinics*, we listed Dr. Ladislav Nagy's title incorrectly. Ladislav Nagy, MD, PD, is the Head of Hand Surgery in the Department of Orthopaedics at the University of Zurich, Balgrist, Forchstrasse, Switzerland. We apologize for the oversight and inconvenience.

# Index

*Note:* Page numbers of article titles are in **boldface** type.

0749-0712/06/$ - see front matter © 2006 Elsevier Inc. All rights reserved.
doi:10.1016/S0749-0712(06)00021-7

*hand.theclinics.com*